DIABETI

Health, weight loss with easy low carb recipes for healthier kidneys

By

EMY SKYE

purposes solely, and is universal as so. The presentation of the information is without contract or any type of guarantee assurance.

The trademarks that are used are without any consent, and the publication of the trademark is without permission or backing by the trademark owner. All trademarks and brands within this book are for clarifying purposes only and are the owned by the owners themselves, not affiliated with this document.

WHY YOU SHOULD READ THIS BOOK

The key to diabetes care and control is managing blood sugar levels. If your blood sugar is not well controlled you leave yourself open to some very serious side effects and related diseases. Parts of the body affected by high blood sugar levels are the eyes, liver, kidneys, heart and later on it will cause nerve damage in the limbs - peripheral neuropathy and damage the blood flow (vascular disease).

The only solution is to regularly monitor blood sugar levels and take action if it is high. It will sometimes blip to a one-off high level but if it is consistently high you need to consult your medical advisor. The remedy will be either a change of medication or modification of your diet or both. As a general rule you should only eat low or medium glycemic index carbohydrates as high index foods produce a very fast rise in blood sugar which will stay high for some time as body of a diabetic does not have the ability to assimilate it quickly like a non-diabetic.

The test is done by using a meter which measures the glucose level in a small sample of blood taken from a finger. Most of the meters use a test strip which absorbs the blood droplet for the machine to analyse. The blood droplet is produced by using a lancet device to make a small incision in the finger. It is best to use antiseptic on the area before and after taking the sample to avoid the possibility of infection.

Sometimes you will find if you are suffering from a cold your blood sugar goes a little high for a few days and this seems to be part and parcel of the cold effects with little you can do about it. If it continues longer than this again medical advice should be obtained.

There are many brands of blood glucose testing machines or glucometers as they are sometimes called on the market but there are 2 main types. The first type is a little more automated and less fiddly where the test strips are kept in a cassette or drum inside the machine and are exposed through a slot when the machine is switched to test. The blood droplet is then transferred to the strip for testing. The second type uses strips stored externally which are inserted by the user into a slot on the machine prior to the test.

Both types of machine take a few seconds to analyse the blood and produce a result on the electronic readout on the machine. Some machines are bigger than others the ones with internal storage tend to be bigger so if you travel a lot and are looking for portability the external strip machines are the way to go.

Having been diagnosed with diabetes, in order to slow down the inevitable complications that are going to arise, you need to start making some changes in your lifestyle. In some cases, those changes could be quite drastic but they will soon be brought into context when compared to the seriousness of acute or chronic consequences that the complications of diabetes can cause.

The absolute key to properly manage your diabetes is get control of your blood sugar levels. This is only possible by regular testing so read on to find out more about it.

People with diabetics benefit from balancing certain food group. in this book we discuss some of the best food to eat, as well as which type to limit

What are the best foods for people with diabetes?

Eating certain foods while limiting others can help people with diabetes manage their blood sugar levels.

A diet rich in vegetables, fruits, and healthful proteins can have significant benefits for people with diabetes.

Balancing certain foods can help maintain health, improve overall well-being, and prevent future complications.

A healthcare professional, such as a doctor or dietitian, can work with people who have type 1 diabetes or type 2 diabetes to find the most beneficial food choices that work for them.

This book looks at some of the best foods for people with diabetes to eat, as well as which foods to limit or balance in the diet.

TABLE OF CONTENTS

INTRODUCTION

Truths About Diabetes

Diabetes has hidden dangers that begin before diagnosis and continue to worsen if certain steps are not taken to prevent the complications that are the true, "killers" in terms of diabetes.

Statistics show that there are around 18 million diabetics in America, both Type 1 and Type 2. It is amazing how many people, diabetics included, who have no idea what dangers a diabetic faces over their lifetime. A diabetic, all things being equal, lives almost 10 years less than their non-diabetic counterpart on average.

Why do diabetics life shorter life spans than non-diabetics? The answer is both simple and complicated. Simple in explaining in general terms, complicated in the medical sense. Without traveling the complicated route in this book, I will try to give a simple, straight forward answer to the above question. Diabetics live shorter lives than non-diabetics because of diabetic complications.

What Are Diabetic Complications?

Diabetic complications are chronic medical conditions that begin to affect the body of the diabetic. These complications are brought about mostly by a condition the medical community had named, "Advanced

Glycation End products" which is simply, "excess sugar" saturating the inside of the cells of the body. This condition also called AGE for short includes coronary artery disease, vascular disease, blindness, kidney disease, retinopathy (blindness) and loss of feeling in the hands and the feet (peripheral neuropathy) among others.

Diabetes in the early stages does not produce symptoms. Unless found during a routine medical exam, it is possible for a diabetic to remain undiagnosed for years. It is during these years that the beginnings of diabetic complications can gain a foothold due excess sugar in the cells (AGE). The statistics show there is the possibility of as many as over 5 million people going about their normal lives while having undiagnosed diabetes.

Are Diabetic Complications A Certainty?

While the current consensus is that the formula for diabetic complications Diabetes + Time = Complications. What this means is there is a much higher potential of a diabetic becoming diagnosed with one or more diabetic complications over time. This is partly due to how well the individual monitors and controls his/her blood sugar.

Drastic rises and falls of blood sugar can be hard on the body and the excess sugar present in the cells create havoc on the different nerves within the body as well as the capillaries, veins, and arteries. The evidence to date show that excellent control of blood sugar and an active lifestyle goes a very long way in preventing and/or slowing down the onset of diabetic complications.

The Different Types Of Diabetes

There are two types of diabetes - Type One and Type Two. Type One attacks children and young adults and is characterized by the pancreas failing to produce insulin which is a hormone that breaks down sugars and starches while converting them into energy. Type Two occurs usually later in an adult's life and is characterized by the pancreas being unable to produce enough insulin due to several factors, obesity being one of them.

Around 10 percent of diabetics are Type One while the other 90 percent are Type Two. The major difference between the two being that Type One diabetics are completely dependent on insulin and take daily injections while the Type Two's have both those who require insulin shots while others can rely on oral medication and/or changes in diet and exercise.

The Risk Factors Surrounding Diabetes

There are several risk factors that can push a pre-diabetic into full blown diabetes.

1) being overweight.

2) family history of diabetes,

3) lack of adequate exercise.

4) history of gestational diabetes (occurs during pregnancy and usually disappears after delivery).

5) certain ethnic groups

People over 45 years of age and has one or several of the risk factors mentioned above should be screened for diabetes each year, preferably during an annual medical exam. It has been shown that people with these risk factors comprise the majority of diagnosed cases of diabetes each year.

What Tests Help Diagnose Diabetes Cases?

There are two, main tests used for determining whether or not a person has a glucose intolerance:

1) Fasting Plasma Glucose Test

2) Oral Glucose Tolerance Test

Both of these tests can determine glucose intolerance which is where blood sugar is higher than what is considered normal. This is not always an indication of diabetes however.

Can The Onset Of Diabetes Be Prevented?

People with the above risk factors can go a long way toward preventing the development of full-blown diabetes by making significant lifestyle change. What are lifestyle changes? Changing unhealthy diets to more blood sugar friendly ones, doing enough exercise to help offset increased blood sugar levels and keep the body healthy and losing weight especially if considered obese by the medical community.

If you are pre-diabetic you need to stay on a strict diabetic diet. Ask your healthcare professional for a diet that meets that criteria and limit cakes, candy, cookies, and other things made of simple sugars. Eat small, nutritious meals and eat 5 times a day instead of only three.

If you are already diagnosed with full-blown diabetes, you should follow the same diet while under the meticulous care of your healthcare professional. Keep your cholesterol, blood pressure and blood sugar within proper limits and have your eyes checked every year.

Diabetes can contribute to blindness, kidney disease and heart disease. Complications caused nearly 70,000 deaths in 2000.

What Can The Diabetic Look Forward To?

Diabetic complications can be prevented or lessened for a longer time period by paying serious attention to lifestyle. A diabetic who eats right, keeps his blood sugar in control and within accepted limits, exercises and gets proper rest can expect to have a quality of life that is much higher in terms of the pain and suffering that diabetic complications brings into the lives of diabetics who do nothing to change their lifestyle.

What begins to occur in the diabetic who starts to develop complications because of uncontrolled blood sugars over time is a life filled with the possibility of becoming an invalid, either blind, an amputee, or suffering renal failure or a heart attack.

The above paints a rather grim picture if lifestyle changes are not adhered to. Research has shown that the diabetic that keeps their blood sugar within acceptable limits and follows a healthy, diabetic lifestyle that has been shown to be effective against diabetic complications stands a much better chance of not developing many of the complications their less than dedicated counterparts do.

There is a new derivative of thiamine (Vitamin B1) available now that is showing great promise in greatly reducing the excess sugar in the cells of the diabetic, the process known as Advanced Glycation Endproducts (AGE).

Before people develop type 2 diabetes, they almost always have "pre-diabetes" -- blood glucose levels that are higher than normal but not yet high enough to be diagnosed as diabetes. There are 54 million people in the United States who have pre-diabetes. Recent research has shown that some long-term damage to the body, especially the heart and circulatory system, may already be occurring during pre-diabetes.

The cause of diabetes continues to be a mystery, although both genetics and environmental factors such as obesity and lack of exercise appear to play roles.

There are two major types of diabetes. Type 1 diabetes results from the body's failure to produce insulin, the hormone that "unlocks" the cells of the body, allowing glucose to enter and fuel them. It is estimated that 5-10% of Americans who are diagnosed with diabetes have type

1 diabetes. Type 2 diabetes results from insulin resistance (a condition in which the body fails to properly use insulin), combined with relative insulin deficiency. Most Americans who are diagnosed with diabetes have type 2 diabetes.

There is also pre-diabetes which is a condition that occurs when a person's blood glucose levels are higher than normal but not high enough for a diagnosis of type 2 diabetes. There are 54 million Americans who have pre-diabetes, in addition to the 20.8 million with diabetes.

Diabetes is a result of problems with the body's ability to produce INSULIN. Insulin controls the amount of glucose (sugar) in the blood and the rate at which the glucose is absorbed into the body cells. The cells need glucose to produce energy. In people with Diabetes, the glucose (sugar) builds up in the bloodstream, instead of being used by the cells for energy. This abnormally high level of glucose in the blood is called Hyperglycemia.

There are two major type of diabetes:

TYPE 1: Affects 5 - 10% of people and normally starts at an early age. Type 1 diabetes sufferers must inject themselves with insulin on a daily basis. These injections are necessary because the insulin (glucose) cannot be absorbed into the bloodstream.

TYPE 2: This is by far the most common form of diabetes and affects 90-95% of sufferers. This type of diabetes usually begins in later years, although, unfortunately, it is now becoming more common in young people. This is caused mainly by being overweight, incorrect eating habits and lack of exercise. Type 2 diabetes is 'life-style' induced. Obesity (over weight) is a major factor in Type 2 diabetes, and weight reduction is often all that is required to control it.

RECOMMENDATIONS FOR DIABETICS

• Change your diet - eat low fat, high fibre, plenty of fruit and vegetables and more fish and chicken. Try not to eat processed foods like white rice, sugar, white maize meal, white bread etc. Do not eat cakes, sweets, biscuits and cold drinks ie Coke. Do not eat convenience foods like takeaways.

• Supplement your diet with Spirulina. Spirulina helps to stabilize blood sugar levels.

• Avoid tobacco in any form as it constricts the blood vessels and inhibits circulation. Keep your feet clean, dry and warm. Because of poor circulation, foot ulcers and sores can develop and once the skin is broken, sores may not heal.

• Diabetes and Blood Pressure often go hand in hand and if you can control the blood pressure problem, this often brings the sugar levels under control.

• 50% of diabetics suffer from Libido problems and the other 50% will experience this problem. This means that all Diabetics will have this problem at some time, and therefore need assistance in this area.

• High glucose levels in the eye can cause damage to the lens - this results in poor eyesight or 'colour blindness'

• Type 2 diabetics (Lifestyle) are less able to recognize sweet tastes and this makes it difficult for them to lose weight. Often this type of diabetes can be controlled by diet and exercise alone.

• Women who have diabetes will find it very difficult to fall pregnant and should start controlling their sugar levels long before she plans to fall pregnant.

• Check your feet every day, try not to walk on rough surfaces barefoot and cut your nails straight across. Remember a small injury can lead to big problems.

Diabetes symptoms may vary from person to person but most of the time anyone with diabetes will experience some or all of these symptoms. Some symptoms are: going to the restroom more often, staying thirsty, fatigue, blurred vision, stomach pain and occasionally people suffer from weight loss.

Type 1 diabetes is normally only found in children and type 2 diabetes is found mostly in adults but not always. There are some cases where children are being diagnosed with type 2 diabetes. Some people may be diagnosed with being borderline diabetic, which normally ends up turning into full blown diabetes but not always.

Some of the most important things people with diabetes should know is a healthy, nutritional diet and a regular exercise program can help in treating the disease. Speak with your doctor about what kind of diet you should consider following, along with a moderate exercise program. The doctor or a nutritionist should be able to tell you exactly what kinds of foods you should be avoiding and give you some tips on how much exercise you need every week. Doing this has many health benefits and will also make you feel so much better about yourself.

You should know the truth about some of the most common myths about diabetes. Myth #1 You can catch diabetes from someone else. No. Although we don't know exactly why some people develop diabetes, we know diabetes is not contagious. It can't be caught like a cold or flu. There seems to be some genetic link in diabetes, particularly type 2 diabetes. Lifestyle factors also play a part.

People with diabetes can't eat sweets or chocolate. If eaten as part of a healthy meal plan, or combined with exercise, sweets and desserts can be eaten by people with diabetes. They are no more "off limits" to people with diabetes, than they are to people without diabetes.

Eating too much sugar causes diabetes. No. Diabetes is caused by a combination of genetic and lifestyle factors. However, being overweight does increase your risk for developing type 2 diabetes. If you have a history of diabetes in your family, eating a healthy meal plan and regular exercise are recommended to manage your weight.

People with diabetes should eat special diabetic foods. A healthy meal plan for people with diabetes is the same as that for everyone - low in fat (especially saturated and trans fat), moderate in salt and sugar, with meals based on whole grain foods, vegetables and fruit. Diabetic and "dietetic" versions of sugar-containing foods offer no special benefit. They still raise blood glucose levels, are usually more expensive and can also have a laxative effect if they contain sugar alcohols.

If you have diabetes, you should only eat small amounts of starchy foods, such as bread, potatoes and pasta. Starchy foods are part of a healthy meal plan. What is important is the portion size. Whole grain breads, cereals, pasta, rice and starchy vegetables like potatoes, yams, peas and corn can be included in your meals and snacks. The key is portions. For most people with diabetes, having 3-4 servings of carbohydrate-containing foods is about right. Whole grain starchy foods are also a good source of fiber, which helps keep your gut healthy.

People with diabetes are more likely to get colds and other illnesses. No. You are no more likely to get a cold or another illness if you have diabetes. However, people with diabetes are advised to get flu shots. This is because any infection interferes with your blood glucose management, putting you at risk of high blood glucose levels and, for those with type 1 diabetes, an increased risk of ketoacidosis.

Insulin causes atherosclerosis (hardening of the arteries) and high blood pressure. No, insulin does not cause atherosclerosis. In the laboratory, there is evidence that insulin can initiate some of the early processes associated with atherosclerosis. Therefore, some physicians were fearful that insulin might aggravate the development of high blood pressure and hardening of the arteries. But it doesn't.

Insulin causes weight gain, and because obesity is bad for you, insulin should not be taken. Both the UKPDS (United Kingdom Prospective Diabetes Study) and the DCCT (Diabetes Control & Complications Trial) have shown that the benefit of glucose management with insulin far outweighs (no pun intended) the risk of weight gain.

Fruit is a healthy food. Therefore, it is OK to eat as much of it as you wish. Fruit is a healthy food. It contains fiber and lots of vitamins and minerals. Because fruit contains carbohydrate, it needs to be included in your meal plan. Talk to your dietitian about the amount, frequency and types of fruits you should eat.

You don't need to change your diabetes regimen unless your A1C is greater than 8 percent. The better your glucose control, the less likely you are to develop complications of diabetes. An A1C in the sevens (7s), however, does not represent good control. The ADA goal is less than 7 percent. The closer your A1C is to the normal range (less than 6 percent), the lower your chances of complications. However, you increase your risk of hypoglycemia, especially if you have type 1 diabetes. Talk with your health care provider about the best goal for you.

There is no cure right now for diabetes but there are several different forms of treatment available for you. Do not give up hope on feeling better and living a long, healthy, happy life. Even if you are one of the many that has been diagnosed with this disease, it does not mean that your life as you know it is over. It simply means you may need medication and you will have to consider certain lifestyle changes that will have an amazing outcome once you have done so. There are many other treatment options that could eventually be available to you but are currently undergoing more detailed research.

What does a lifestyle change mean to a diabetic? Well, usually the first response is, "You want me to do what!" Which is closely followed by, "What's that?" Next usually comes, "Well, if I can't have everything I like to eat anymore, have to start exercising everyday and begin taking medication all the time, what's the point of living?"

Well, guess what! It's a sure bet that if you don't start making all those changes in your life NOW, you won't be living a quality life for much longer plus you'll be taking a chance on letting a whole lot of other really bad things go wrong with your body!

Ask any diabetes specialist whether people can begin to control their diabetes through diet and exercise and the answer will be a resounding YES! It has been proven in studies all over the world time and time again.

The key to making this change is having the patient make a conscious committed decision to change all their old habits. They must then begin implementing the new changes in small steps into their daily lives until they have replaced the bad habits with the new habits, which in turn equals a new lifestyle.

A new lifestyle just means changing habits-natural eating habits, a habit of getting up and moving for at least 30 minutes each day, stopping a smoking habit, reducing an alcohol consumption habit. All of this has to be done not for just a few months but for a lifetime in order to get this silent killer under control.

Another added benefit of changing your lifestyle is lowering your blood pressure and the risk of a stroke or heart attack, less sleep apnea and more vim and vigor for a better life overall. This change must become a way of life for you, for your whole life, not just for a few months or a year.

Your life literally depends on it.

Sure, there will be slip-ups now and then but you just have to shake it off and get started again. Don't beat yourself up over it. It will be easier to begin again the next time because you've been there before and know what went wrong and how you can regain control. Just think about feeling and looking better and avoiding all the possible diabetic complications in store for you if you don't change.

But the best outcome of your new lifestyle will be the plus of being with your loved ones as a healthy person years longer.

What does a lifestyle change mean to a diabetic? Well, usually the first response is, "You want me to do what!" Which is closely followed by, "What's that?" Next usually comes, "Well, if I can't have everything I like to eat anymore, have to start exercising everyday and begin taking medication all the time, what's the point of living?"

Well, guess what! It's a sure bet that if you don't start

making all those changes in your life NOW, you won't be living a quality life for much longer plus you'll be taking a chance on letting a whole lot of other really bad things go wrong with your body!

Ask any diabetes specialist whether people can begin to control their diabetes through diet and exercise and the answer will be a resounding YES! It has been proven in studies all over the world time and time again.

The key to making this change is having the patient make a conscious committed decision to change all their old habits. They must then begin implementing the new changes in small steps into their daily lives until they have replaced the bad habits with the new habits, which in turn equals a new lifestyle.

A new lifestyle just means changing habits-natural eating habits, a habit of getting up and moving for at least 30 minutes each day, stopping a smoking habit, reducing an alcohol consumption habit. All of this has to be done not for just a few months but for a lifetime in order to get this silent killer under control.

Another added benefit of changing your lifestyle is lowering your blood pressure and the risk of a stroke or heart attack, less sleep apnea and more vim and vigor for a better life overall. This change must become a way of life for you, for your whole life, not just for a few months or a year.

Here are some lifestyle tips for the healthy diabetic-

1. Change your diet.

A healthy diet coupled with proper nutrition can help the diabetic manage his or her condition. Obese people are at more risk to diabetes. So it is very important for diabetics to maintain a healthy weight. Actually, it is not only the diabetics who need to eat healthy. Changing your diet to healthier alternatives can help prevent other diseases in the long run. It is essential for the diabetic to especially cut down on carbohydrates, because glucose comes from this food group. And diabetes is concerned about the erratic levels of glucose in one's body. The amount of fats and salt one takes in should also be controlled. Diabetes has some associated risks including high blood pressure and high cholesterol. Healthy eating can simply help in minimizing these associated risks and prevent any more diabetic complications.

2. Lead an active lifestyle.

Being sedentary is the worst thing a diabetic can do. Daily exercise can help a diabetic lose weight and maintain it at healthy levels. As mentioned earlier, diabetes has some associated risks like high blood pressure and high cholesterol.. Exercise can lower bad cholesterol levels and raise good cholesterol levels. Exercise also lessens stress levels of the body. Another benefit of exercise is that it releases endorphins which are the natural pain relievers of the body. Exercise makes the blood circulate normally which is sometimes constricted due to the high glucose levels coming from diabetes.

3. Monitor your glucose levels constantly.

Glucose testing on a constant basis can help the diabetic monitor his or sugar levels and make adjustments on their food and medicinal intake. A diabetic who does not know how to check up on his or her glucose level is like a beginner driver mindlessly maneuvering a vehicle. It is definitely imperative that a diabetic knows how to test his or her glucose level. This will aid the diabetic in controlling his or her food intake. This will also warn the diabetic if his or her physical activities are not enough. All diabetics have a mark or goal on what their glucose level should be. Testing constantly can help diabetics in managing properly their condition.

Diabetes should not be life sentence. With discipline, a diabetic can lead a healthy and happy life. The above lifestyle tips are simple enough for the diabetic to follow. Constant encouragement from family and friends can help the diabetic achieve this healthy lifestyle. Except for constant glucose testing, the said lifestyle tips are actually applicable to everyone. And apart from for gene-influenced diabetes, diabetes can actually be prevented. Even people without this condition should be aware of the above lifestyle tips in order to prevent going into the other direction.

If you or someone you love has diabetes, it's important to get educated. Diabetes is very treatable, but requires knowledge and care.

CHAPTER 1
ACHIEVE HEALTHY WEIGHT LOSS

Weight loss happens when a person is in a state of negative energy balance. This means that the body is losing more chemical energy during work than it is gaining from food or other nutritional supplements. This means that it will essentially use up the reserves of fat that are stored inside the body to fuel the processes that it needs to fulfill the everyday operations that it needs.

For people who are already at a healthy and medically acceptable weight, they might want to lose weight for the purposes of improving athletic performance or simply to meet weight classes in a particular sport. Boxing and wrestling are just a couple of examples. For other people, they might want to lose weight in order to shape their body into a more attractive physique.

For some people, the term weight loss has been associated with mental conditions such as bulimia or anorexia. For the medical community, unintentional weight loss is not healthy and may certainly be a precursor to a more significant condition such as a poorly maintained case of diabetes mellitus. But in general, losing weight is a good thing especially if you are planning to do it to increase your fitness level. This type of weight loss is a good thing because it will generally improve one's fitness, health as well as appearance.

For individuals who are on the heavy side or obese, therapeutic weight loss will certainly decrease the chances of that individual from developing the dreaded disease of diabetes. Those people who are overweight and obese also run the risk of developing other health conditions such as high blood pressure, osteoarthritis and coronary heart disease. The list will go on and on and the detrimental conditions that one can develop over time is simply too staggering to fully weigh. If one would want to undergo an effective and health weight loss program, it should be noted that a physicians should be asked first. This is because a physician will be able to accomplish a specific weight loss plan that will be custom-made for the person. This is important because the weight loss methods or program that a morbidly obese person might not work on you since you might probably be eating the same amount of calories that you are consuming as of the moment. If you try adapting a weight loss program that is geared for someone else, you run the risk of following the wrong method.

For those people who are already afflicted of the disease of diabetes, it would be very ideal to consult with a specialized physician who can offer specific advice in order to trim down your weight to an ideal level. The American Diabetes Association has actually studies proving that through a combination of a strict diet and exercise program, the ADA has found, a 5-10% loss of body weight will produce a 58% reduction in diabetes.

This is an excellent fact that may spur any diabetes patient to lose the necessary number of pounds that may affect them.

You should begin your safe and healthy weight loss journey by considering your own needs There's no one diet program that will be best for everyone.

Start by assessing any emotional or physical conditions that might interfere with your weight loss. It's best to see your physician.

You'll find that the majority of experts will recommend a healthy eating plan and regular physical exercise for healthy weight loss.

Adequate amounts of vitamins, minerals, and protein (recommended daily allowances) should be considered for including in any weight loss plan. Your plan should be lower in calories, but not in these essential elements.

Its well known that the body requires a certain amount of vitamins and minerals to function properly and remain healthy. A healthy diet can supply your body with the vitamins and minerals it needs. Problems and disorders will almost certainly arise if your diet is not supplying your body with these essential elements

Everyone who wants to shed weight will tell you that they want healthy weight loss. Unfortunately, only a handful can actually tell you how to clearly define it. Healthy weight loss is achieved if you fulfill the following principles.

Firstly, you have to make sure that all of your weight

loss comes from losing fat. In other words, the total weight that you reduce comes from losing only fat and nothing else. Many people think that they are losing only fat when they reduce the number on the weighing scales but this is proof of their ignorance. You can also lose a lot of water and muscles in the process. At times, you could even be losing more water and muscles than fat. This is very harmful to the body. In summary, healthy weight loss requires that you lose only fat and the least amount of water and muscles.

When you lose weight healthily, you will boost your metabolism instead of suppressing it. This is very difficult to achieve with your conventional fad diets which almost always suppress your metabolism. Excessive muscle loss is the main reason for a suppressed metabolism. Losing weight healthily requires that you incorporate strength training into your lifestyle. This helps to build your muscle mass and keep your metabolism high.

When all of your weight loss is the result of fat loss, you will enjoy enhanced health. This is because the process of building muscles and losing fat naturally balances your hormonal system. You will have lower cortisol and insulin levels. Both cortisol and insulin are potent fat storage hormones. You will have a higher level of potent fat burning hormones such as the Human Growth Hormone and testosterone. Health is also tremendously enhanced when you carry a lower amount of body fat. It puts lesser strain on your heart and the other body organs.

You do not enjoy the same amount of health enhancement if you had lots of muscle and water loss. This is typically what happens when you focus on losing weight. The excessive loss of muscle tissue reduces your strength, worsens your posture and makes you susceptible to falling or injuring yourself.

When all the above conditions are satisfied, you would have lost only fat and not much muscles and water. You will enjoy enhanced health. The fat loss will be sustainable. All these results are only achievable if you have incorporated regular exercise and a healthy diet as a part of your lifestyle. When all this has been achieved, you can be sure that the weight that has come off, will stay off. This is the definition of healthy weight loss.

Consuming the incorrect type of meals and bad eating habits is the root cause of being over weight. Cultivating good eating habits by understanding when to eat and what to eat is the first step to a healthy weight loss diet.

Typical knowledge has us consuming three meals a day. Nevertheless the secret to any successful and weight loss diet is to eat 5 meals a day. That way the body is able to enhance its metabolic rate that can burn fats faster and effectively.

In any healthy weight loss diet ample dietary consumption of carbohydrate, protein, fats and water is crucial.

1. Carbohydrates

Better known as carbs for short, are sugars and its most important function is to supply the body with energy. It is stored within the liver and muscles and are referred to as glycogens. Too much intake of carbs will force the glycogen to turn into fats.

In any healthy weight loss diet eating the best carbs is essential. There are two types of carbs namely low-glycemic and high-glycemic carbs. Low-glycemic carbs releases glucagons into the body and utilizes fats for energy source. High-glycemic carb meals consists of baked potato, french fries, sugar sweetened beverages, sweet bars, sugar and others raises the amount of glycogen levels in the body that turns to fats.

Eat the proper carbs to avoid weight gain is the first dietary guide in any weight loss diet program.

2. Protein

Protein aids in the improvement and repairing of muscles, red blood cells, hair tissues and generates a healthy immune system.

Consuming excessive protein meals is an effective healthy weight loss diet that accelerates the development of muscles within the body that will increase the metabolic rate and burns fats faster.

Diet should include egg white, fish, meat, poultry, milk, vegetables and seeds.

3. Fat

Fat have been given a bad reputation for years as it's at all times related to weight gain. Nonetheless fats are vital for the formation of cell membranes, manufacturing of hormones and primary energy needs.

Figuring out what kind of fat to eat is essential in any healthy weight loss diet.

Eating good fat like mono-saturated fats helps cut back LDL cholesterol level. Meals such as cashew nuts, almonds, avocados, virgin olive oil, pistachio nuts are well balanced wholesome weight lost diet foods.

Polyunsaturated Fats, Omega three and Omega 6essential fatty acids, are needed by the body as it is unable to provide them by itself and is obtainable from our diet. They're essential in brain development, stopping coronary heart disease, lower high blood pressure and improving HDL. Good cholesterol level and maintain bone health. Healthy weight loss diet ought to embody fish such as salmon and tuna, kiwifruit, walnuts and hazelnuts, meat and others.

Trans Fatty Acid stands out as the worst fat that may be consumed. It is counter productive to any diet because it will increase the LDL (terrible) cholesterol level and reduces the HDL (good) cholesterol level. Trans fatty acid are present in butter and processed foods.

4. Water

Water is a necessary part of a healthy weight loss diet. It helps transport nutrients all through the body, regulates the body temperature and aids in digestion.

Water should be made a part of a health weight loss diet as it helps to burn fat because:

a. the body will automatically retain and store water in

the cells thus increasing body weight if it lacks water. As soon as there is sufficient water then the stored water will be released into the body system.

b. without water the kidneys are unable to function efficiently and the liver has to help. Due to this fact it is unable to burn as much fats thus storing them within the body instead. Drinking loads of water will free the liver and burn the fats.

How to Choose a Healthy Weight Loss Regimen

Are you looking for a healthy weight loss program that truly works for you? Choosing the right plan is no mean feat. With all the products, plans, and promotions that are out in the market today; it is quite hard to distinguish which ones won't jeopardize your health. What are the key things to remember to make sure that you're choosing a healthy weight loss plan? Here's a quick rundown of the main factors to consider in deciding what comprises a truly healthy weight loss plan.

Stay Away from Single-Item Diets

Most of us have heard of The Grapefruit Diet, The Cabbage Soup Diet, and The Twinkie Diet. Any diet plan that encourages you to eat from only one food source spells trouble. Though these meal plans might help you lose weight during the first few days, they are merely temporary solutions. Single-item diets do not provide the proper nutrition your body needs to function properly, nor do they pass as healthy options. Starvation means depriving your body with essential nutrients, making it an instant recipe for failure. Healthy weight management allows you to eat food that promotes fat loss and lean muscle growth without the need to starve yourself.

Find a Program that Computes your Calorie Intake

Find a healthy diet plan that provides a specific calorie intake that will allow you to lose just the right amount of weight each week. It is recommended to lose no more than 2 pounds a week. This is an achievable goal. By being mindful about your caloric intake, you'll soon see your pounds go down. The key to losing weight the healthy way is a slow and steady approach. There is no such thing as instant. Remember that you've gained weight through time, and you'll have to lose weight through time too. If you religiously follow a healthy weight loss plan that breaks down calories into fat, carbohydrate, and protein; you'll be surprised to know that you can still eat food while losing weight.

Consider Portion Management and Water Intake

Portion control plays a key role in any weight management. A truly healthy diet plan makes you feel hungry before each meal. It also teaches your body to distinguish between being hungry and being full. In addition, drinking lots of water is recommended as it helps induce satiety during meals and promote hydration. These are all essential in healthy weight loss. Water is also vital in detoxification which helps eliminate water weight gain.

Time to Get Active, Slowly but Surely

A healthy weight loss plan provides a good balance of healthy diet and exercise program. Start engaging in a physical activity for 20 minutes at least thrice a week to enhance your metabolism and support your healthy weight loss goals. Keep it simple at first and just put all your energy in gradually increasing your heart rate as you progress overtime. To achieve your ideal weight, choose a healthy regimen that you can easily stick to until you reach your desired weight.

Be mindful of all these characteristics when choosing a healthy weight loss plan. Always remember to value proper nutrition above all else, and weight loss should naturally follow.

Permanent Weight Loss Equals Healthy Weight Loss

Permanent and healthy weight loss can not only improve ones self-esteem, but it can also be an integral part of increasing overall physical, mental, emotional and spiritual well-being. However, many weight loss approaches train the victim (You!) to do all the wrong things, and eat all the wrong foods, leading to rebound weight gain. If you lose weight in a healthy way, then you weight loss will be permanent.

Weight Watchers Damages Metabolism

I have seen so many people going to a program like Weight Watchers completely ruin their metabolism by losing more muscle than fat. They get applauded every week when they improve their weight loss by losing muscle. In the long run, this person ends up gaining the weight back because of the metabolic slow-down due to the loss of muscle, which is discouraging to say the least.

Diet and Detox Weight Loss

No healthy detox weight loss plan is complete without a well-balanced diet of REAL FOOD! I recommend a colorful Mediterranean diet that is modified to be low glycemic index. Establishing a healthy diet does not mean taking away all carbs; nor does it mean stocking your shelf with low-fat diet foods. Rather, you should intake a diet full of lean proteins, plenty of non-starchy vegetables, and limited amounts of beans, healthy fruits and nuts. Optional would some limited amounts of whole grains. Of course, no detox diet would be complete without plenty of pure water.

Movement and Detox Weight Loss

In addition to a nutritious diet and plenty of water, movement is also important for detox weight loss. Regardless of what type of movement you enjoy, the important thing is to get going! Try walking five times a week for about 30 minutes. Not only are you getting exercise and burning calories, but you are also moving lymph, and stimulating blood flow through your tissues - essential for proper detoxification.

If you live in a northern climate where walking outside might be dangerous in the winter due to slippery conditions, most malls welcome exercising walkers. If walking is not your thing, consider becoming a member of the local gym. There are typically many cardio options such as bikes, elliptical machines, stair stepping machines, treadmills, etc. In addition, most gyms offer weight machines, free weights, balls, etc. Most gyms also offer classes such as spin classes, aerobics classes, and more.

If you have to chose between cardio and resistance, the science shows that you will burn more fat with in the long run with resistance exercise, especially if you do large compound movements that work large muscles in groups, spiking your heart rate. This high-intensity approach will boost your metabolism for over 48 hours. So doing both resistance and aerobic exercise is best, but rest assured that a simple 150 minute a week walking program along with a scientifically-based detox diet weight loss plan will work

If you just can't seem to go it alone, an investment in a personal trainer may be worth your while as you try to achieve some healthy fat burning. Though personal trainers may seem expensive, they can often prevent injuries by making sure you use the proper form.

I know that an injury may be a far-off thought for you right now, but trust me, an injury can really set back your weight loss and belly fat reducing goals dramatically. Imagine not being able to exercise at all! Rather than exerting maximal effort, the better choice is to dial it back a bit to prevent injury. Train don't Strain is the watchword

Diet Pills Are Crap

You know from reading my diet pills book than 99.99% of the diet pills out there are pure crap! The only diet pills that actually work without a rebound effect are ones that nourish the detoxification pathways of the body, so the liver gets decongested and fat is burned faster. You will see a lot of other benefits too, digestion improving, skin and eyes getting clearer, rashes and skin conditions spontaneously clearing up, and aches and pains going away. The best side effect of including detox nutrition in your fat-burning plan is this: When you are toxic, your body retains a lot of water. When you detox and diet at the same time, you lose that extra water weight quickly, without dehydrating yourself, accelerating your slimming and weight loss. In this case, the water loss is healthy, because it is not from using diuretic diets pills, but occurring naturally from having healthier, less-toxic cells.

Fad Detox Diets Increase Toxicity and

Impair Fat Burning

Fasting on only fruit, the "Master Cleanse", the "Popcorn Diet" and other unhealthy fad detox diets really all fall down for two reasons:

First, your body needs a wide range of nutrients to be able to detoxify and excrete toxins. When you are on a super restricted mono diet or fad like the Master Cleanse, you actually impair the detoxification process, impeding your fat burning!

Second, toxins and their toxic metabolites circulate in the body and get redeposit in the tissues causing toxicity headaches and flu-like symptoms. Unknowing consumers of the fad detox diets frequently assume that their headaches, body-aches, and runny noses are a sign that their fad diet is working; but in fact this indicates that they are missing critical nutritional substrates for proper detox.

I cannot emphasize enough how unhealthy these fad detox diets are. They both impair fat-burning and detoxification and increase toxicity.

A Healthy Detox Diet Approach

Though there are many weight loss methods out there, but for best results we recommend a healthy detoxification diet approach that includes movement, an eating system for life, and plenty of tissue cleansing nutritional support for speedy results. A detox diet for life means a non-fad detox diet that supplies you with the protein, fiber, and other nutrients to nourish healthy body structures and metabolic detoxification pathways so your body can detox every day, for the rest of your life.

When your goal is detox weight loss, then apply these same principles with reduced caloric intake, and consider supplementing your healthy whole-food detox diet with a scientifically-based supplement that nourishes the metabolic detox pathways for enhanced results.

While everyone understands that being overweight, or obese, is "not good for you", many people do not understand the risks they and their loved ones face if they fall into this category.

Obese or overweight people are at increased risk for some or all of the following conditions:

1. Various forms of heart disease

2. Strokes

3. Diabetes

4. Cancer

5. Arthritis

6. Respiratory problems

7. Psychological disorders

6. High blood pressure or hypertension

It is estimated that 300,000 deaths in the U. S. each year are associated with obesity, and the economic cost of obesity in the United States was about $117 billion in 2000. Economic costs include the out-of-pocket expenditures of the individuals involved, the costs of the institutions and organizations which help provide services, and the costs borne by every member of society whether they are in this group or not.

A healthy weight loss program could do much to help individuals avoid the personal and financial risks associated with being overweight while helping them achieves longer, happier, more productive lives more years of healthy enjoyment once they leave the work place behind them.

Unfortunately these days, one is more likely to hear of a "fast" weight loss program than a healthy weight loss program, and it is next to impossible to include both terms in the same sentence. The fast weight loss programs which are so prevalent are short term, temporary "fixes" when they fix anything at all. These programs, which commonly involve drinks, supplements, pills, or exotic exercise equipment, simply do not work, at least not for permanent, healthy weight loss.

Worse, many of these fast weight loss programs may actually contribute to further weight gain, decreased enjoyment of life, diminished health, and, in extreme cases, even death.

Fortunately, there are healthy weight loss programs, plans, systems, and options which can provide, or contribute not only to healthy weight loss, but a lifetime of healthy weight management.

While a full program would take a book to explain all the possible actions you can take for healthy weight loss, here are a few tips that can help anyone get started on a lifelong program for health and fitness.

Here are some tips on how you can lose those unwanted pounds the healthy way:

1. Start moving. One of the most effective weight loss strategies around is exercise. Sadly, many people have no idea how much or which exercise they should do. Many do not even realize that simple, enjoyable activities such as gardening, swimming, or playing tag with the kids can be part of an exercise program. Exercise is such a diverse topic that anyone serious about losing weight should do a little research on the types of activities that may possibly be a part of their weight loss program.

2. Eat smart. There is a lot you can do to improve what and how you eat, but some of it takes training and knowledge most people do not have. It also involves all sorts of convoluted decision making, sometimes based on charts and lists, good carbs, bad carbs, high glycemic index foods and low glycemic index foods. If you are able to learn all that great, but just use come common sense in the meantime. Eat lots of veggies and fruits, have some protein, but not a ton, and stay away from stuff with sugar. Teach yourself to use artificial sweeteners instead of sugar, and start looking at labels.

3. Eat small. Eat small, healthy meals and snacks several times a day. One failure mechanism built in to a diet is the denial of food. It is not just the denial of pleasure of food and eating, but your body also reacts one way when food is denied, and another when it is regularly supplied daily with small healthy meals and snacks.

4. Team up. Get together with a friend who has much the same goals as you. Take a walk with them every day. Meet them for lunch. They won't make faces when you order something for your health rather than for the fun of it. In fact, why not get a group together? That way, if one person is not available, maybe someone else will be. Plus the social interaction is good for you. People who "go on diets" tend to start avoiding people, and that often is at least a part of the reason they fall off the diet wagon.

5. Think health. Don't try to lose weight. Instead, try to get healthy. First of all, a positive goal is easier to work towards than a negative one. Second, doing things to make yourself healthy is easier to sell to yourself and to others than "trying to lose weight". Also, there will be setbacks along the way. These are normal. If you fail to lose weight as fast as you think you ought to, or if you gain weight, in your mind you will have "failed". If however you eat a second piece of pie, you have slowed down on your path to health, but you can get back on track within minutes simply by going for a walk or remembering to use sweetener in your drink rather than sugar.

6. Get rest. When your body is tired, certain chemical changes take place and substances are released that contribute to weight gain or slow weight loss. It is easier to get involved in activity when you are rested.

7. Have fun. Two of the reasons you want to lose weight is so that you can feel good, and feel good about yourself. You want to enjoy life. It works both ways. If

you lose weight and feel healthy, you will want to enjoy life, and you will feel good about yourself. If you go out of your way to enjoy life, you will probably be more active, and this, combined with other beneficial effects related to weight gain and weight loss will help your healthy weight loss program.

8. Drink water. Many times we interpret the body's signals as hunger when they are actually thirst. Often, a glass of water will satisfy what we believe are hunger pangs. Keeping the body properly hydrated helps it process toxins and perform a myriad of functions more efficiently.

9. Don't quit. When you are on a healthy weight loss program, your weight loss will be slow. Many people are disheartened when they think of only losing one or two pounds a week on average. However, that would be a weight loss of 52 to 104 pounds in a year and 104 to 208 pounds in two years! To put that in proportion, I had a friend who had a gastric bypass. She was told that even with surgery, she would probably only lose about 75 pounds in her first year, and the weight loss would slow down in the second year! Many people could accomplish similar results just by building up to a daily 20 to 30 minute walk and by cutting a few empty calories out of their diet.

By the way, if you have not been exercising and begin exercising as part of a healthy weight loss program, it is highly likely that you will actually GAIN weight at first. Don't let this dishearten you. It is entirely normal and can actually be considered part of the body's preparation to lose weight and live a healthier life!

Be happy with your results. If you are living in a healthy manner, you will lose weight. Certainly, how much weight you lose will depend on a lot of factors, and, if you are walking 20 minutes a day and haven't lost what you would like to lose, you can walk 30 minutes a day, or 15 minutes twice a day. Adapt and move on. However, do not expect to be the man or woman you were in high school or college. You might never fit into your old prom dress or army uniform again. I don't, and I exercise regularly and try to eat right. I feel great and am in excellent health, but my old army uniform is just a memory hanging in my closet now.

Go on. Have some fun. Do what you can. Reward yourself for your gains and forgive yourself for non-gains. I refuse to call them failures. There is no failure until you give up completely.

CHAPTER 2
SAFE AND HEALTHY WEIGHT LOSS FOR DIABETICS

Healthy living should always be an option as opposed to anti-hypertension medication. High blood pressure is a major contributor to other serious medical issues such as heart attack, stroke, kidney failure or heart failure. It has been proven that weight loss and blood pressure are interrelated; therefore one of the most effective ways to take control of your health is to loose weight.

Basically, your blood pressure rises as your body weight increases. The more pounds that you are over your desired body weight will increase your chances as a candidate for high blood pressure. Obesity affects over 60 percent of adults in the United States alone.

Even as it is difficult to understand the complexity of it all, the general relationship between weight loss and reduced blood pressure is the ultimate change in lifestyle. Consequently, a modification in systolic and diastolic blood pressure is proportionally related to the amount of weight loss.

It is always beneficial to monitor your blood pressure at home between visits to your physician. If you are aware that you are not within your desired body weight, it is important that you take precautions and adopt a healthier lifestyle. A healthier diet will help you prevent and control high blood pressure.

When you are overweight, losing just ten pounds can lower your blood pressure. Not only is overweight and obesity major risk factors for high blood pressure, it may also induce the development of high blood cholesterol and diabetes, which are also risk factors for heart disease. There are two key elements that determine if you are overweight or obese; body mass index (BMI) and waist circumference.

The BMI is the measure of your weight and its relation to your height. This element gives an approximation of your total body fat. Subsequently, this body fat increases the risk of diseases that develop due to obesity. Because the BMI cannot fully determine risk in some cases, such as body building or edema, the waist measurement is also taken. Too much body fat in the stomach area also increases disease risk. Specifically, any woman that measures more than 35 inches in the waist or a male that measure more than 40 inches is considered a risk.

The key to losing weight is simply calorie restriction. You must eat fewer calories than you exert in daily activities. Physical activity is extremely significant when considering the advantages of weight loss and blood pressure. In addition to consuming fewer calories, weight loss also requires salt intake restrictions, especially for people who are already victims of elevated blood pressure.

Once you have succeeded at weight loss, be sure to

maintain your healthier lifestyle regimen. Loose the weight by implementing regular exercise and substantial nutritional guidelines. It is crucial that you understand the relation and importance of weight loss and high blood pressure.

Losing weight as a diabetic can be very efficient and easy. You must work as a team with your nutritionist and doctor. Also, keep in mind that nothing happens overnight, so the results may not actually be visible until after a few months (3 - 5 approximately). Every drastic diet, with huge weight loss in a short period of time, has side effects, and one of most common one is known as the yo-yo effect (when you get back all lost weight, after only few weeks).

Diabetics weight loss also includes eating healthy, exercising, drinking a lot of fluid (water and natural juices) and if possible - taking some products and supplements which will help you burn fat and improve your metabolism. If you are a diabetic, you know how important it is to control your weight, and live stress free. That is why we have created a checklist for you; to help you stay healthy and get fit fast!

First of all, make a doctor appointment. Your doctor can give you advice on how to lose weight healthy and without risking or ruining your health. Weight loss for diabetics is not a taboo, it is not a problem and it is not a health issue. But, you still need to talk to the specialist before going on a diet. Doctor will help you lose weight healthy and without stressing your body.

If you are serious about losing weight, a doctor is not the only person you need in your corner. A dietician is also a crucial part of your weight loss plan. She will set weight loss goals with you, and help you create a menu while on diet. Eating healthy is half of the job. Weight loss for diabetics excludes every possible carbohydrate diet. These diets are not suitable for you because they can have a terrible impact on your blood sugar. Always keep this in mind, this is for your own good.

Exercise at least four times a week. The gym is a good solution but if you don't have enough time then cycle, walk the dog, instead of driving - walk around. Jogging is also a very useful part of weight loss for diabetics. Tennis comes in handy too, and so does basketball. Find your ideal activity and go for it. Soon, you will be amazed with good results. During your weight loss process monitor the level of glucose in your blood as often as you can. It would be good if you can do that 2 or 3 times every day. If you see any changes, contact your doctor as soon as possible.

Eat smaller portions but more often. Instead of having two or three large meals, eat 5 or 6 times a day, but smaller portions. Also count your calories, and drink a lot of water - at least 1l every day. This is much healthier, helps you stay full during the day and prevents hypoglycaemia. Weight loss for diabetics must be supervised by a doctor! Keep that in mind and start eating healthy, exercising and feeling better.

If you plan to lose weight by going on a closely monitored diet, you have to make sure that you have the right sugar levels because weight loss for diabetics, especially when done through a specific diet can be a lot different from those that normal people can have. Choosing the right food to eat can be very crucial for diabetics because it could mean a matter of life and death for them.

If you have diabetes it is very important for you to know that your illness is a condition in which your body has excessive sugar that your body cannot use. It generally comes from sweet and starchy foods. Starchy foods can be bread, rice potatoes and a lot more. Sweet foods are those that have high sugar content like chocolates, ice cream and cakes.

With these facts in mind, it would be reasonable to say that you should avoid those foods. Although most doctors would not let you get rid of them totally, it would still be best not to take foods that are rich in contents that could trigger your illness. If you would like to lose weight effectively and at the same time be in perfectly good health, it would be best if you consult your doctor or a registered dietician. They know best what foods you should be having that would be able to supply your body all the essential vitamins and nutrients without putting your health at risk.

Weight loss for diabetics does not have to be hard especially now that there are already alternatives for the foods that you cannot have. Like for example if you are craving for a sweet dessert, there are now sugar alternatives available for diabetics that can be purchased at any drug store. If you would like to have an ice cream, you can already satisfy your craving because there are already available ice cream alternatives for diabetics and they do not make you fat because they do not have sugar or have very limited calories and carbohydrates.

For a lot healthier living, you can ask your dietician as to what fruits and vegetables you should best have. You can choose to have those that contain the least amount of calories, sugar, carbohydrates and other fatty substances.

It is also a must for any diabetic to drink at least eight glasses of water everyday to make sure that the excessive fats and other impurities in the body are washed away. Other than controlling your food intake, it would also greatly help you to effectively lose weight if you do some exercises that will be able to help you get your body in shape. Losing weight should not be hard for you especially if you can manage to do some effective and simple physical exercises.

Many diabetics are overweight. This is no coincidence, overweight people are bound to have blood sugar problems if they remain overweight for a period of time. Weight loss for diabetics is the primary goal to get control of a diabetics blood sugar levels. Whether you are type 1 or 2 you can get control over your diabetes just by losing 5 to 10 % of your body weight. Even if you only lost 5 to 10 lbs you could see a drop in your blood sugar levels. Being overweight and not eating healthy will have a negative impact on your blood sugar.

Choosing to eat healthy foods is important for anybody's diet but for a diabetic it is even more important.

Diabetic complications can be life threatening so eating right and losing some weight to control or postpone your diabetes should be on top of your list.

When you decide to take action and find a healthy weight loss for diabetics program your goal should be able to lose weight while keeping your blood sugar levels in the normal range so you do not have to take as much medication. A good weight loss diet for diabetics allows you to lose the weight that contributes to the very health problems that you are facing now.

A good starting point to all those with diabetes is to take a look at the food pyramid at the American Diabetes Association website.

A weight loss for diabetics diet should be low in saturated fat, cholesterol, and simple sugars. You should be eating green leafy vegetables and fruits in moderation due to the high sugar and starch contents. And incorporate plenty of whole grains high in fiber.

Also a weight loss program for diabetics needs to incorporate protein from lean sources that are high in omega 3 such as fish.

As type 2 diabetes rapidly increases with the current rate of obesity, weight loss for diabetics is becoming something that many diabetics need to be looking into. It is especially important for diabetics to learn to control blood sugar levels by effectively losing weight. Start your losing the weight today that may have you off insulin in time and free up your life.

Is there a healthy weight loss system for those

suffering from type 2 diabetes? One might ask, and the answer is yes. Healthy weight loss for diabetics will require a more careful approach than your regular weight loss enthusiast, but aside from close monitoring of the blood sugar and constant check-up from your doctor, everything should be the same.

Most of type 2 diabetics are constantly monitoring their blood sugar levels making this reminder somehow pointless. But stressing the need and importance of this reminder, it is very crucial that along the way of your weight loss program, you must regularly check your blood sugar level, as cutting out on some portion of the regular amount of food that you consume, and most physical activities have direct effects on your sugar level and of course your health.

Your diet has a direct effect on your health and mood due to the rising and lowering of your blood sugar level, so make it a point to consult your doctor before taking any weight loss diet program. There are a lot of diet system out there that have successfully worked for other diabetics, which has also done convincing results for them.

One such diet system that has been strongly helping type 2 diabetics with their weight loss is the Nutri System. This dietary system offers restaurant grade foods that are high on good cholesterol, great for managing blood sugar levels. The best thing about this is that meals are delivered on to your doorsteps at the time of specification, so you don't need to worry about not getting nourished on time.

Cardio vascular activities which may come in aerobics, brisk walking, running or yoga, have direct effects in lowering your blood sugar level. These exercises will make you better able to control your blood level and the best thing about adding exercises to your weight loss program, it that it allows you to eat more. Instead of burning 600 calories a day, just put it on 300-400, the important thing about it is your managing of your blood sugar.

As oppose to the immediate lowering of blood sugar level with cardio vascular exercises, heavy weight training will tend to spike sugar levels when you least expect it, say for example, when driving your car. Make it a point to check your blood sugar before getting in your car, on your way home from the gym. You can also bring some power bars on the way.

Consulting with your doctor, as important as it is, may come only when you feel that along the way for health loss program is working against your health. Doctor consultation will be better and will work at your advantage, before starting something new with your program, like diet shifts and new workout routines.

Healthy weight loss for type 2 diabetics is possible and doable. The most important thing to be done, is to keep a close monitor of your blood sugar levels every time possible, to be in the safe side. Of course get approval from your doctor at the start of any programs that you will undertake, be it diet or exercise.

CHAPTER 3
DIABETIC MEAL PLANNING

Diabetics think about food a lot. Under other circumstances, this obsession with food could be considered unhealthy. However, most diabetics come to think about food in a healthy way - as fuel for the body. Diabetics must come to terms with eating as a means to provide the body with energy. Many diabetics have come to realize that diabetes may actually have saved their lives. These individuals find that they experience a period of rigorous diabetic meal planning followed by a diabetic lifestyle based on what they have learned.

Diabetic meal planning involves two major aspects - education and advice. An educated diabetic is better equipped to assist in the planning of his or her treatment plan. Diabetics are also offered advice from several sources that include health care providers such as a doctor or registered dietitian in addition to other diabetics. Your initial visit to a registered dietician will probably provide you with more information than you can digest immediately. You may find that joining a self-help group of diabetics will help ease the education and management of your diabetes. For any diabetic, the first course of action for managing their diabetes is diabetic meal planning.

At first, diabetic meal planning can be a daunting task.

As a recently diagnosed diabetic, you may find that planning your meals takes more time and energy than you are used to - and it probably does. The days when you just grabbed a meal on the go without really thinking about the effects that what you were eating was having on your body are gone. Now you will be living a lifestyle that must promote healthy eating.

Diabetic meal planning really is meal planning. You will not merely be thinking about what you will be eating. You will be writing your meals down. You may even want to keep a food diary at first. A food diary will help you identify potential trouble spots in your diet. Taking your food diary with you to your appointments with your dietitian or to your diabetic help group meetings may help you receive valuable input into your diabetic meal planning. Use all of your available resources to help you with your diabetic meal planning.

Gather as many recipes and free diabetic meal plans as you can and take them with you to your appointments or group meetings. Solicit the advice of seasoned diabetics when planning your own diabetic meals. Your dietitian in addition to other diabetics are the most valuable resources when considering your own diabetic meal planning. A registered dietitian is best able to help you with the nutritional aspects of your meal planning and other diabetics can help you with the realities of living with diabetes. Your diabetic meal planning will not only have to provide you with a diverse menu for make-at-home meals, but it will also have to be flexible enough so that you will know what to eat when you are on the road.

The recipes and meal plans you have gathered will consist of valuable information as well as throwaway advice, but you will definitely find that you have learned from both the good and the bad. Combining what you have learned into your own comprehensive plan is what diabetic meal planning is all about. Determining what is right for you, considering your own personal preferences, lifestyle and caloric needs, is your own individual road map for managing your diabetes. Once you have navigated the wealth of information out there for you to take advantage of, you will be left with what is, for you, the best path for a healthy diabetic lifestyle.

Diabetes has entered your life with a bang. Perhaps you know others who are diabetics, perhaps not. Perhaps you have friends or family members who are diabetic. Perhaps you were secretly expecting diabetes to strike, perhaps it came as a surprise. You are now faced with some important choices - first and foremost, your diet.

Any diabetic must think and plan his or her meals. This planning becomes second nature in time and will not always be as overwhelming as it may seem when you are newly diagnosed. Since the majority of diabetics suffer from Type II diabetes, or adult onset diabetes, you have likely had poor eating habits for some time now. You will now need to take some time to educate yourself and to actually sit down and write out your menu.

One of the first people that your diagnosing physician will direct you to will be a registered dietician. Your dietician will help you in planning your meals and will likely provide you with recipes for healthy eating. You will go over your own individual diet needs. Each diabetic is different. You may need to lose weight in addition to managing you diabetes. You may need to gain weight in addition to managing you diabetes. Your lifestyle will have a bearing on what your diabetic needs are. Diabetics with active lifestyles have different caloric needs than those who lead relatively sedentary lives. Your dietician will consider all of these factors and then will assist you in developing a diabetic diet sample from which you will determine the meal plan that is right for you.

With the wealth of information that is now available via the internet, diabetics have many resources right at their fingertips. Diabetics are no longer limited to the information that they are given. Diabetics are encouraged to find as much information as they can about their condition. Education is the key to living a healthy diabetic lifestyle. Many reputable diabetes organizations have internet web sites and most of them provide surfers with a diabetic diet sample. Many of these web sites have forums on which you can network with other diabetics that can offer more diabetic diet samples. Diabetics today have more information available to them than diabetics did just a decade or two ago.

A well-planned diabetic diet sample will take the reader through at least one day of planned meals. Using what will likely be the diabetic food pyramid, the diabetic diet sample should include food exchanges and how to use them. Using an example, the diabetic diet sample will build meals based on a number of exchanges to clarify the method that a diabetic will use to create his or her own meals. A diabetic diet sample may also include recipes that are based on food exchanges. Cooking a stew, for example, may include exchanges from several different food groups. You may use meat exchanges, vegetable exchanges, and fat exchanges to create a stew or casserole. Meals based on a combination of exchanges may seem difficult at first but will soon become second nature. Keeping your diabetic diet samples and your diabetic recipes close at hand will give you the tools you will need for a successful diabetic diet.

Arm yourself with as many diabetic diet samples as you can access. The more samples you have the more food choices you will have to begin with. Until you become familiar with the process of creating meals from you allotment of food exchanges, let these diabetic diet samples will be your guide. Don't' worry at first about creating your own meals. Once you are comfortable with planning your own recipes and meals, you will find that you can share your own diabetic diet samples with other newly diagnosed diabetics.

Diabetic Weight Loss Diet Guidelines

Here are the 4 rules, weight loss for diabetes management that will interest you.

1. Reduce Snacking by keeping yourself busy. Construct a daily plan without having too much free time. This way you keep out of the kitchen for a quick snack, whenever you are free. And if you absolutely must snack, be choosy. Go for snacks such as unsalted nuts, dried fruit

unsweetened, fresh fruits and vegetables and dark chocolate. What's easy diabetic weight loss principle isn't it?

2. Increase of fruit and vegetables in your meals as fresh fruits and vegetables contain vitamins and minerals essential for health of body, Susan proposes to introduce more of them as part of a diabetic weight loss menus.

3. Consume more water, 8 cups a day for a healthy diet. Even though it is a statement a decade old, it still rings true. Water clear toxins from the body and cool the temperature of the body. According to experts dehydration can make you hungry. Drinking water before a meal can suppress hunger. For the ladies there is more motivation to drink more water. It makes you look younger, because water hydrates the skin. The advantages are almost limitless. Drinking water is a necessary activity in your diabetic weight loss regime.

4. Select the entire Meal carbs, instead of white flour to remember this recommendation is if you can't remember the rest. Following this rule, Susan was able to lose much weight. Indeed, other diabetic friends lost her weight, successfully keeping only the rule alone.

By the way, here's tip for the entire meal with choice of product: where it is possible to go for fresh one without preservatives or added ingredients. Basmatic and brown rice are excellent choices and so the whole meal pasta. When unwanted pounds melt away, applying these simple changes, you agree that your journey for diabetic weight loss is simple.

Diabetes Diet Guidelines

Diabetes is proving to be one of the most frightening diseases I've ever had but easy to manage so far. Over the past 6 years I've done very well controlling my Type 2 Diabetes with a healthy diet and exercise, the lack of which having been the cause of my problem in the first place. I'm not a doctor and don't play one on the internet so don't do anything in this article without checking with yours. But, because it seems so difficult at first, I want to share with you some things I've discovered which simplified the whole diet thing for me.

Diabetes Diet programs are everywhere, but many are so severe or so complicated we can't follow them. When my doctor diagnosed me, he gave me a copy of a typed diet sheet that really took all the joy out of my life...no sugar, bread, rice, cake, ice cream...etc. Fortunately, he sent me to a diabetes diet class which taught me you don't have to give up sugar or other carbohydrates...all you have to do is manage them. That's made all the difference! In fact, to manage Type 2 Diabetes, all we have to do is eat the balanced diet we should have been eating all along.

The American Diabetes Diet recommends we get 50-60% of our calories from carbohydrates, 12-20% from proteins, and less than 30% from fats. In my personal diet, I lean toward 50-30-20% in those groups. As you can see, 50-60% carbohydrates isn't exactly eating none...is it? We'll get into easy ways to mange this balance later. I found the biggest dietary adjustment I had to make was taking 3 big meals a day and turning them into 3 small meals and 2-3 snacks. This is necessary to keep a balanced level of blood sugar (glucose). The funny thing was, after about a week, I noticed I had more energy and never felt hungry. Needles to say, I started getting excited.

Eat Generally Healthier: The smallest adjustment was to eat healthier...you know the drill: More fresh fruits and vegetables, more fresh meat, fish and poultry (lean cuts) and less fruit juices and processed foods. More crackers and fewer chips. More whole grain breads and pasta and fewer white, processed flours. More brown rice and less white. Low or non fat milk, cheese, yogurt, salad dressings. Eat cakes, cookies, pies, ice cream, sodas, etc. less often and preferably low fat, sugar free varieties if possible. The amazing thing to me was, there was literally nothing I couldn't eat...I just had to control the way I ate. This isn't as hard as people think.

Make it pretty easy to classify your foods and know how much of each you should be eating. Here are some general classifications to get you started. Fats include butter, margarine, oils and nuts. Proteins include meats, fish, poultry, eggs, milk and cheese (milk and cheese are high in fat). Carbohydrates include bread, cereal, beans, grains and potatoes. Sugars are refined carbohydrates and should be taken in very small amounts. Almost all fresh vegetables are "free" because they are high in fiber and nutrients without being high in fats, carbs, etc. All packaged foods have labels that tell you how large a serving is and how many carbs, sugars, proteins, fats, calories are in a serving. This is more important to read than the price.

Portion Size is easy to figure for foods. If you learn the exchanges and portion sizes for given foods you never have to count carbs, calories, etc. Just look at what you're eating. Here's a little chart to get you started:

A serving of… Measures… And is about as big as…

Cheese - 1 ounce - Four dice.

Rice - ½ cup - Half a baseball.

Bagel - 4 ounces - A hockey puck.

Meat - 3 ounces - A deck of cards.

Peanut butter - 2 Tablespoons - A ping-pong ball.

Pasta - 1 cup - A tennis ball.

A Simple Diabetes Diet Guideline: I manage my diet using exchanges and portion control without measuring anything. I've found each day I can balance my diet and keep my blood sugar normal by managing my portions as follows: 5-6 Carbs, 5-6 Proteins, 5-6 fruits and vegetables (mostly vegetables), less than 3 fats, and 2-3 quarts water. Make sure to include high fiber foods in your fruits and vegetables to help maintain good blood fat and sugar levels. I lost about 50 pounds in a year and maintained it for 5 years since the onset of my disease. I'm now starting to lose the last 40 pounds toward my goal of 180. That's really about it! Of course, you'll want to study as much as you can and ask you doctor to fully manage your diabetes, but I hope this chapter has removed some of the mystery and given you a good starting point to take control of your diet. You can do this!

CHAPTER 4
WHY A LOW CARB DIET MENU IS THE BEST FOR WEIGHT LOSS

For many years, eating a low fat diet was the ticket to losing weight. After all, fat has 9 calories per gram, and carbohydrate has only 4 calories per gram.

A whole range of low fat foods hit the market: low fat cheese to use on pizza, low fat pasta sauce for paste dishes and low fat margarine to butter your toast and sandwiches...

Yet our waist line got bigger not smaller, and the more we chased the low fat diet, the fatter we got. Why?

Essential fatty acids found in foods such as extra virgin olive oil, seeds, nuts, avocados, and oily fishes such as salmon and mackerel are actually good for weight loss. The unhealthy fats, or trans-fatty acids of partially hydrogenated fats such as margarine and processed fast foods are the ones to avoid.

For the past seven years, ever since a study in 2002 concluded that dietary fats were not a contributor to weight gain, the focus has shifted to carbohydrates and sugars.

Unfortunately, our society is bombarded with foods containing an excessive amount of carbohydrate. A subway anyone? How about McDonald's with fries and a shake? Pizza night? Pasta? Sugary cereal?

Topping the Glycemic Index (GI) foods list at 80 or over are:

French baguette (95), Lucozade (95), Baked potato (85), Cornflakes (83), Rice Crispies (82) and Prezels (81) to give a few examples. Glucose is obviously 100.

So if you are having sugary cornflakes for breakfast, a French baguette sandwich for lunch and baked potatoes for dinner, you are overloading your system with too much carbohydrates, and your chances of losing weight is looking a bit grim.

On the lower end of the GI scale at under 40, we have:

Apples (38), wholemeal spaghetti (37), chickpeas (33), dried apricots (31), kidney beans (29), lentils (29) and cherries (22) to name a few.

So why is a low carb diet menu so important for weight loss?

When you consume an excess or a large amount of carbohydrates, you body kicks into overdrive and delivers a large dose of a hormone called insulin to deal with all the excessive carbs. This large dose of insulin tends to convert the starch and sugars into fat.

The resulting high blood sugars in your body will also

mean the body is using carbohydrates as energy, rather than fat. Plus what it cannot use will be converted into more fat. The result? The fat stays and more gets added with each high carb intake.

Eating a low carb diet will mean your insulin level will be on a more even keel. A high fiber, low GI meal will satisfy your hunger more and help control your appetite. Your body will also start using fat as energy (provided you are not a total coach potato!).

A note on snacking....

Healthy snacking is good for you. It will stop you from eating excessive amounts at meal times and will maintain a more balanced level of blood sugar. Numerous studies have shown that eating smaller meals more frequently helps weight loss. You will feel less hungry and the quantity you eat will be smaller.

Healthy snacks would include fruit, nuts and vegetable.

Finally, a low carb diet does not mean a no carb diet. Just limit your intake of bread, cereal, pasta, rice, potatoes and other high GI foods, and you will be well on your way to a healthier weight.

Instead of carbohydrates being the center of the dish, make protein and vegetables the main items. Just use carbohydrate as the side condiment, (a bit like the token decorative vegetables you get in restaurants) and not as the main dish.

Think "low carbohydrate", not "no carbohydrates" and

you will be on your way to losing weight and getting healthier.

CHAPTER 5
HOW DOES A LOW CARB DIET WORK?

L ow carbohydrate (or low carb) diet plans have really increased in popularity in the last ten years or so. This is in large part due to the success of the ever-popular Atkins diet and the low carb diets that followed it such as the South Beach diet. But you don't need the latest book or high priced diet program to follow a low carb diet. All you need is some basic dieting knowledge and one of the many low carb free diet plans that can be found on the web.

Low carb diets are typically low in carbohydrates (duh!) and high in fats and proteins. How low the carbs are supposed to be depends on the particular diet plan. Typically, low carb diet plans start you off for a week or two of very low carbs. Meals typically consist of meat (lots of meat!) and vegetables with some zero carb sauces or dressings; no dairy, grains, or fruit allowed. Then certain carbs are slowly added to the meals but never at a high percentage. Typically, carbs will account for 5% - 20% of your calories on a low carb diet.

Why low carbs? When you eat carbohydrates it raises your blood sugar level. This in turn causes your body to release insulin. It is insulin's job to get that sugar (glucose) out of the bloodstream and into your cells. First it tries putting glucose into muscles and when the muscles are full of glucose insulin pumps the remaining glucose into fat cells. While the insulin is doing its work your body will burn the glucose in your bloodstream first before trying to burn your fat. So, if you can keep the glucose level low in the bloodstream, insulin won't put that glucose in your fat cells and the body has very little glucose in the bloodstream to use for energy. Therefore, the body must use something else, like fat, to burn for energy. This is the theory behind low carb dieting.

So now that you know the basics of low carb diets you know what to look for when searching for free low carb diet plans on the web or diet books in the bookstore. The low carb diet plan should steer you far away from starchy carbs like white bread, white rice, and pasta and encourage you to eat leafy green vegetables to get the fiber, vitamins, and minerals your body needs without spiking the glucose levels.

One final thing to take into consideration is that a low carb diet totally goes against the USDA's food pyramid guidelines. Although low carb diet plans are popular modern science has not determined whether they are healthy or not. There are issues with the increased levels of fat consumption (particularly saturated fat consumption) and it's effect on cholesterol in a low carb diet. You should do the research and check with your doctor to see if low carb diets are right for you.

So the question is, will a low carb diet be an effective tool to lose weight?

The answer is a resounding YES!

It is one of the best tools and most effective methods of shedding weight fast. There are a few points that must be followed for a low carb diet to be effective.

First, we need to understand what a diet is. A low carb diet program is a program that restricts the consumption of carbohydrates. The percentage of carbs consumed should not exceed 20% of caloric consumption for the day.

Fats and protein will make up the rest of the calories. Fruits and vegetables are allowed on a diet. The harmful carbs however, are kept to a minimum.

What are harmful carbs?

Food with sugars and white flour such as donuts, pasta, white bread,etc, white rice and potatoes. These are considered as high glycemic foods that spike your blood sugar levels.

When you avoid these foods, you will not gain weight fast and your body will not have insulin spikes. In fact, avoiding these foods will prevent health problems like diabetes.

You should be consuming healthy carbs in moderation for the low carb diet to work effectively. Low carbs does not mean no carbs. Many folks make the mistake of avoiding carbs completely.

This is wrong. You must consume carbs of the healthy variety.

Vegetables and fruits are healthy carbohydrates. You

may also wish to switch to carbs with a lower glycemic index. Instead of eating white bread, you can opt for whole grain bread. Switch white rice for brown rice.

So why does a low carb diet work so effectively?

The reason that a low carb diet works so well is due to the fact that most people consume the wrong kind of carbs. They eat white bread, pasta, etc. What these carbs do is that they cause spikes in insulin and blood glucose levels.

These indirectly lead to fat storage, increased appetite and sudden hunger cravings. The cravings lead to overeating of these same carbs and the vicious cycle continues.

By eating carbs with a low glycemic index, your blood sugar and insulin levels will stay constant. You will feel full and satiated for a longer duration. You will also not have sudden cravings for unhealthy food or an unexplained increase in appetite.

Being on a low carb diet has several health benefits. These have been proven through studies that have been conducted for the past few decades.

A low carb diet will give you more energy. Contrary to popular belief, a low carb diet will not leave you feeling sluggish. You will experience mental clarity too. Your joints and body will be less painful.

Bad carbs tend to cause inflammation in the body. This could explain why many people constantly feel aches and pains in their joints and muscles. Their body is suffering from inflammation.

These are just some of the benefits that have been reported by those who have embarked on a low carb diet. It is highly recommended that you adopt this diet permanently even after you have reached your desired weight.

Once you reach your desired weight and know how many calories you should consume daily for maintenance, then you can allocate 20% of those calories for healthy carbs and you will maintain your figure for a long time.

Because a low carbohydrate approach to weight loss is a relatively recent trend (growing in popularity over the last twenty years), and because it challenges many more traditional ideas about safe and healthy ways of losing weight, you may be wondering if it is actually going to be good for you to embark on a low carb diet plan. Also, because to maintain weight loss you need to commit to restricting the amount of carbs you eat for the rest of your life, you probably want to know if it is healthy to make that sort of lifestyle choice.

You can actually get all the nutrients and energy you need from a low carb diet. If you think about it, before the invention of farming techniques and mass food production, people used to live only on what they could hunt or gather. There was no way of processing cereals to turn them into food, and before people could cook there was no way to eat naturally occurring starchy foods like potatoes.

Humans, like most mammals, are designed to be able to manage this kind of diet very well. This is why the body stores fat in the first place, it is a good fuel to keep in reserves in the body. Of course, now that food is abundant in the Western world, most of it in some way processed, most people take on more "fuel" than they need, and the reserves of fat end up being bigger than we would like them.

By sticking to a low carb plan, you often end up eating a lot of whole foods, such as meat and vegetables, rather than processed foods, because those are usually full of carbohydrates. This is a much more natural and beneficial diet.

Also, because on a low carb diet your blood sugar levels stay stable and constant, you feel healthier and more energetic, and you will be far less likely to develop diabetes.

You may ask how a diet that is high in fat can ever be considered healthy, because excess fat can damage the heart and cause all sorts of problems and complications, however actually, on a low carb diet, dietary fat is not a problem. This is because when you are on a low carb diet your body uses fat instead of carbohydrate as its source of energy, and so the dietary fat you consume gets used up very quickly. If you were to eat that much fat while consuming carbs too, your body would use the carbs as its primary fuel source, and the fat you ate would stay in your body. That is when it causes problems (and of course weight gain). Fat without carbs is perfectly fine - you have to have one or the other to keep your body going.

Basically, switching to a low carb diet is a healthy option for most people, however if you are concerned or you have other health problems and you are worried you may not be compatible with low carb living, speak to a doctor.

CHAPTER 6
IS A LOW-CARB DIET RIGHT
FOR DIABETES?

If you've recently been diagnosed with type 2 diabetes, you've probably been hearing a lot about carbohydrates. Out of the three primary macronutrients in food -- protein, fat and carbohydrates -- it is the carbohydrate that your body most easily turns into blood sugar.

It's a well known fact that the more carbs you eat, the higher your blood sugar will become -- and the more insulin your body will need to keep your blood sugar levels in check. Because of this, numerous studies have focused on whether a low-carb diet is actually best for keeping diabetes under control, and the resounding answer appears to be yes.

What Does the Research Say About Low-Carb Diets for Diabetics?

A study by Duke University Medical Center researchers found that after 24 weeks on either a low-carbohydrate ketogenic diet or a low-glycemic reduced-calorie diet, obese people with type 2 diabetes fared better on the low-carb regimen. Those following the low-carb ketogenic diet:

Had greater improvements in hemoglobin A1C (a measure of blood sugar control)

Were more likely to reduce or eliminate their use of diabetes medications (95 percent of the low-carb study participants did so)

Lost more weight

Cutting carbohydrates from your diet has a double benefit for diabetics in that it not only causes your blood sugar levels to go down, it also helps you lose weight, which is also beneficial for blood sugar control.

A ketogenic diet, which is high in fat and very low in carbohydrates, is often used to help control seizures in people with epilepsy and also sometimes as a weight loss tool.

Normally when you eat, the carbohydrates you consume are turned into glucose, but when your diet is very low in carbs and high in fat, your body will burn fat for fuel instead. This leads to the production of ketones, which replace glucose as the energy source. Since glucose is not highly metabolized on a ketogenic diet, it essentially blocks the damaging high glucose metabolism.

A similar study by Swedish researchers also revealed that obese people with type 2 diabetes had improvements in blood sugar and weight loss while following a low-carb diet. Further, those who were insulin-dependent were able to cut their daily dosage in half. As with the previous study, the benefits were derived from a diet in which carbohydrates were very limited, in this case to just 20 percent of their total calorie intake.

Even after 44 months, a follow-up study revealed lasting results.

Yes, Your Diet Can Reverse Diabetes!

Acceptance is growing among the mainstream medical community that type 2 diabetes is reversible. One of the primary ways to achieving this is by modifying your diet, and specifically by modifying your diet to limit carbohydrates.

Despite this, the American Diabetes Association generally does not recommend very low carbohydrate diets, not because they aren't effective but because they believe most people will not stick with them in the long run. It does take some adjusting to cut most carbs from your daily meals, but a primary motivation for doing so is the potential to cure your disease. If you need motivation, remember that staying away from carbs may mean that you can also eliminate insulin, diabetes drugs and even diabetes from your life entirely.

All Carbs are Not Created Equal

When you start out limiting carbs from your diet, it's important to know which carbs need to be eliminated. You're still going to be eating some -- perhaps 20 percent of your food intake or more will be from carbs -- so you've got to choose them wisely.

In the Swedish study noted above, carbohydrate

consumption was limited to vegetables and salads. Refined and starchy carbs like bread, pasta, potatoes, cereal and rice were avoided, and this is a very good model to follow.

If you have type 2 diabetes, it's very important that you avoid refined carbohydrates, which are found in bread, pasta, cereal, cookies, candy, cakes, soft drinks and desserts, as these have been clearly linked to obesity, insulin resistance and type 2 diabetes. In fact, research has shown that the more refined carbohydrates you eat, the more likely you are to develop type 2 diabetes.

So what types of carbs should you eat?

The kind in fresh, non-starchy vegetables. These are the carbs that will actually help lower your risk of diabetes. One study even found that eating green leafy veggies like broccoli, kale, spinach, sprouts and cabbage each day lowers your risk of type 2 diabetes by 14 percent.

At the Functional Endocrinology Center of Colorado, we generally recommend that patients eat four times the amount of vegetables as protein, as this allows you to easily incorporate plenty of health-boosting veggies into your meals without worrying about measuring portion sizes.

The key to remember is that as you incorporate healthy carbs from non-starchy vegetables in your diet, you need to reduce those from other sources like bread, pasta, sugar, rice, cereal and white potatoes.

Low Carb Diets and Diabetes

The low carb craze is here and it looks like it will be staying. What does this mean for diabetics? Low and reduced carbohydrate diets may be able to help diabetes control their blood glucose levels without the use of medications or insulin. In addition to blood sugar control, low carbohydrate diets have been shown to reduce the risk of heart disease, increase energy, and promote weight loss.

Note: Any person who is taking medication or is under the watch of a health care professional should talk to your health care provider before starting any new diet regime. Note 2: Very low carbohydrate diets are dangerous to Type I Diabetics.

How Low Carb Diets Work

Low carbohydrate diets reduce the easiest used form of fuel for the body, carbohydrates, to a degree that the body uses its own fat reserves for fuel. Keeping the protein, fat and nutrient intake constant and high, the body keeps from cannibalizing vital tissues to obtain proper nutrition. Breaking down fat for fuel is called ketosis. Dr. Atkins gives a very thorough description of ketosis in his series of books. This biological process is vastly different from starvation ketosis and ketoacidosis. In starvation ketosis, the body is receiving little to no food at all and begins to break down fat, muscle, bone, and organs to keep itself alive as long as possible. In ketoacidosis, a condition nearly exclusive to Type I

Diabetics, the body begins to break down itself to obtain any usable energy, even if there is sufficient glucose in the system or food intake. This was the main cause of death in Type I diabetics before the discovery and practical use of insulin.

How Low Carb Is Done

Most low carbohydrate diets are similar: restrict the amounts of carbohydrates you intake and you eat nearly anything else unlimitedly. But wisely, the level of restriction varies. In Dr. Atkins' book, he suggests 20 carbohydrates per day, during phase one as directed by a physician trained in low carbohydrate eating, then ramping up the carbohydrates during phase II until weight loss nor weight gain is happening (phase III) and remains there for the lifetime of the client. Other plans state a 30 to 40% of total intake of food be carbohydrates as the single phase to be done indefinitely. There are also numerous variations between these two extremes. Two factors that remain constant are that processed foods, sugar, and processed oils are unhealthy and fruits and vegetables are to be the most important part of the diet. All also go on to say that if a person goes back to the unhealthy habits that caused the health problems or weight gain, the health problems or weight will return. Most plans assume people will remain on the plans indefinitely and rarely mention yo-yo dieting on low carbohydrate diets, since it is not healthy in any case.

What's the best way to do Low Carb

The best way is under the care of a physician specifically trained in low carbohydrate dieting. For those who want to do it themselves, my suggestion is to read up on the research in low carbohydrate dieting and the various types of diets. Anyone can begin by cutting out processed foods, added sugars, and trans-fatty acids. This alone will give tremendous health benefits. A meeting with a nutritionist or physician will give better insights on other foods to add to your diet.

In a low-carb diet plan, the carbohydrate consumption is restricted to between 5 to 10 percent, such that healthy protein and also fats (Like Coconut Oil) take precedence in one's eating practices, to be able to remain satisfied also stay clear of food cravings. It remains in keeping that sensation of fullness that people have the ability to prevent the desire for sugary foods, as well as this is a good factor for diabetics to take on a diet plan that is reduced in carbs to manage their problem. Following this type of diet plan protects against extreme usage of carbs, which causes greater degrees of blood sugar level.

Diabetic issues is a problem where the physical body is not able to effectively absorb carbohydrate as well as sugar. For a diet plan to operate in support of a diabetic, it needs to be reduced in fat, rich in fiber, as well as had with minerals, vitamins, phytochemicals, and also anti-oxidants. Keeping to the sort of food with reduced glycemic index is likewise crucial. Foods that are allowed in low-carb diet plans are meat, chicken, eggs, cheese, fish, as well as some chosen veggies.

Although some resources claim that to remove carbs entirely is not suggested for diabetics, as carbs in the diet plan are important, due to the fact that they act as the primary source of power as well as nutrients within our physical bodies. In a diabetic's diet plan, carbs in too high quantities could be opposed, yet authorities suggest an everyday dose of not less than 130 grams. On the other hand, researches have actually revealed that the low-carb diet plan induced no unfavorable results on the levels of insulin, sugar, blood stress or cholesterol. It is additionally rewarding to keep in mind that people could change a diet plan saying his/her certain demands. Here, prior to adhering to any type of diet plan, make certain to get in touch with your doctor making certain you will certainly be getting all the best nutrients that will certainly aid you to manage your problem. Doing this will certainly help aid you to identify parts of the program that you maybe change for a better eating habit.

The impacts of restricting the quantity of carbs in your diet plan are shown as loss of weight as a result of a lower calorie consumption, or the effective upkeep of your optimal weight. Keep in mind that with weight-loss, the physical body's blood glucose as well as insulin degrees normally boost. Also merely a 10 percent weight-loss is a significant renovation in the direction of remaining in far better control of diabetic issues.

When weight loss is your objective and getting into much better health and wellness makes your problem much more acceptable, after that a very carefully prepared diet plan is ideal coupled with a workout plan that is very easy s to comply with. Daily walks as well as a number of load repetitions with barbells excel low-impact workouts you could start. Normal a workout does not just assist battle with diabetic issues; it likewise adds a feeling of wellness that helps you keep the best perspective to living a much healthier life permanently.

The benefits of Coconut oil... Coconut oil is basically a free fatty acid. It is a medium length compound. What that means is it is used by the body a fuel and not stored as fat in the tissues. 1 Tbs (tablespoon) of coconut oil contains 120 calories. That's as much as 8 tsp (teaspoons) of sugar. The difference is that the sugar is stored as fat. If you are looking for a good oil for cooking or baking or weight loss. Look no further than Coconut Oil. If you want to weigh 125 pounds. You need to maintain 1875 calories a day. Any more you gain weight. Any Less you lose weight. When using coconut oil DO NOT count the calories into your daily intake. They are FREE calories. Long length fatty acids like olive oil, corn oil and even lard is much harder for the body to digest. The calories that are not burned by the body is stored as fat.

Not all carbs and fat are created equal. In the case of Coconut oil you get the best of both worlds. Yes it is a fatty acid. Yes it does contain 120 calories per Tbs. But being a medium length fatty acid your body uses it as a fuel for energy not stored as fat like most fats.

How Low Carb Diets Help Diabetics

Since diabetics need to control their blood sugar, controlling the sugar intake is the easiest and safe route to take. Since Low Carb diets automatically reduce the carbohydrates and hold it steady over the long term, diabetics have an easier time controlling the fluctuations in blood sugar. Once the blood sugar/insulin balance becomes stable, the body usually begins to heal itself, further reducing the need for artificial insulin.

Using a Low Carb Diet For Diabetes

Most doctors and many people with diabetes think that diabetes is mainly managed by changes in insulin doses or tablets. Diabetes may indeed be controlled with tablets or with insulin but diet is absolutely fundamental in long term well being as well as in glucose control. Many people with diabetes can achieve excellent control by dietary means alone.

In the early days diabetes was seen as all about sugar - simply a disease of blood glucose and so a low carbohydrate diet was the obvious and standard advice. We now know that diabetes is far more complicated than this, and the treatments are designed not just to keep blood sugar levels down, but to prevent the complications that occur over the years. We have to take in our calories in some form and if we reduce carbohydrate we must increase protein or fat. Even lean meat, rich in protein, contains quite a lot of fat. People with diabetes are at increased risk of heart disease and it has been accepted for many years, despite a lot of evidence to the contrary, that a high fat diet is bad for heart disease. Therefore the advice from organisations such as the American Diabetes Association and Diabetes UK has been to use a diet low in fat and rich in "complex" carbohydrates.

Complex carbohydrates are said to have a low glycaemic index because they release glucose slowly. Sugars have a high glycaemic index as they release glucose fast. Even foods with a low glycaemic index are likely to lead to a significant rise in blood glucose levels, although the rise will be smaller than with those having a high glycaemic index. High peaks of blood glucose should be avoided. They seem to be toxic to cells and may be responsible for causing many of the complications of diabetes including coronary artery disease.

The whole question of the supposed dangers of fats in the diet is beginning to be looked at again, and the pendulum is swinging back towards cutting the amount of carbohydrate in the diet. Average blood glucose levels are reflected in the concentration of glycosylated haemoglobin (HbA1C) in the blood. Lower levels are associated with fewer complications in both Type 1 and Type 2 diabetes. But some people think that it is the fluctuations in the levels which matter just as much as the averages. It is not yet clear whether the source of the problem is fluctuations in glucose or insulin levels - both may be involved.

Low carbohydrate diets are at least as effective for weight loss as low-fat diets. Weight loss is important for those who are overweight as it reduces resistance to insulin. Substituting fat for carbohydrate has been shown in many studies to be beneficial in terms of weight loss and in reducing the risk of heart disease. Weight loss itself leads to better control in diabetes, but the benefits of a low carbohydrate diet are greater than those just connected with weight loss and are also seen in people with diabetes who are not overweight.

For many doctors, low carbohydrate diets are still controversial but the evidence supporting this approach is growing. Some people have reported "cures" for diabetes using very low carbohydrate diets, but these diets tend to be unpalatable and few can tolerate them. It may be that weight loss and improved blood tests might be due to the combination of an increased protein intake together with restriction of carbohydrate, but this is not yet clear. Higher protein intakes reduce glucose production from the liver and minimizes the excessive secretion of insulin, and people on diets higher in protein or fat eat less because these lead to a greater feeling of fullness and satisfaction.

As the advantages of lower carbohydrate intakes in diabetes are becoming increasingly accepted, the major associations and doctors' organisations are beginning to change their recommendations, but the rate of change is slow, and people with diabetes are starting to take matters into their own hands.

As you may be aware, some doctors support low carb diets while others do not. Consider a situation where you have a doctor that does not believe in them. Typically, they will tell you to eat a "normal" amount of carbohydrates, and then take medications or insulin to compensate for what you body cannot do on its own. This actually leads to weight gain, and can create unhealthy eating habits. Oddly enough, you may not even realize that target weight goals are being shifted upward each year. This happens mainly because the average number of obese people continues to go up. In the meantime, these shifting values make it very hard for a diabetic person to fit into the "average" population.

Individuals that make use of low carb diets tend to follow a very different pattern. Among other things, they often require little or no medication. Some may never need insulin as long as they are able to keep their blood sugar at an acceptable level. Contrary to "regular diets", people that use low carb, or restricted carb diets tend to lose weight. As may be expected, this is an added bonus for anyone that is obese, or suffers from heart complications.

In general, you should not plan to cut all carbohydrates from your diet. As long as you balance your meals, your carbohydrate intake may not need to be slashed below a healthy level. For example, if you consume 1,000 calories per day, you should be able to get by with 120 - 150 grams of carbohydrates. If your blood sugar levels are within normal limits, then you can increase your caloric intake, and adjust your carbohydrates accordingly.

Diabetics that want to go on low carb diets often feel like they cannot talk to their doctor about it. In these situations, some simply go out and start reading books and assembling their own diet. While this initiative is to be commended, you also need to make sure that you are getting the right information. This will be very hard to assess if you cannot speak with a doctor that understands how low carb diets work. When it comes right down to it, lowering your carbohydrate intake can be extremely dangerous. If you do not work with a doctor that is amenable to guiding you in the right direction, it can cost your life.

Many people with diabetes are frustrated with endless adjustments to medications, buying expensive foods, and dealing with nonstop monitoring. Even though their regular doctor may not recommend low carb dieting, there is plenty of information on this topic. You will also find that some doctors will actually counsel you on how to reduce your carbohydrate intake. In order to find this type of physician, you can simply look in the yellow pages of your phone book, or make a few calls to doctors listed in your insurance plan book. Without a question, if you believe this type of diet can help you, then you should make it your business to find a doctor that will listen to you and work with you.

CHAPTER 7
TIPS FOR A DIABETIC DIET PROGRAM AND EATING SENSIBLY

Certainly eating correctly in compliance with your diabetic diet program is essential. Eating nutritious wholesome foods and living a healthier life is a significant part of living with diabetes. Changing your life style is essential as a person suffering from diabetes; life style change can prevent cardiovascular complications that may kill you out right if left neglected.

If in the past you have been eating unhealthy foods and this has led to you gaining unwanted weight, there are numerous eating plans which have originated in response to this particular unhealthy problem.

Consume more food items and shed weight - The main element to accelerating your metabolism is eating a lot of little meals. Eating sweets and certain foods with highly processed sugars needs to be given up absolutely, since they increase blood sugar levels considerably.

Consuming fewer calories than your current body mass index requires will slow your metabolic process and result in an increase in weight instead of a weight loss. Experiment with lowering and increasing your calories you consume and the calories you burn off by taking exercise until you discover a strategy that works for you.

Eating to lose weight naturally - Many individuals associate reducing weight with being gloomy and hungry, however, you can easily eat healthier whilst still dropping those unwelcome surplus pounds. A wholesome, low-calorie diet regime may well make you feel much more satisfied and full of energy. Making it possible to tackle long-overdue jobs or undertake a brand new hobby. Consume mainly real foodstuff - meats, seafood, eggs, reduced fat dairy items, salads, fresh vegetables, fresh fruits and whole grain products.

Eat reduced fat healthy foods - This really is incredibly easy because of the low-fat choices offered in supermarkets and health food store. (Check labels) Eat five to six small meals a day, such as a lot of nutritious carbohydrates, so that you continue to be satisfied and alert together with uninterrupted glucose levels during the day. Excess weight surrounding your tummy comes with a heightened overall health risk - follow a healthy eating plan and obtain that ideal shape.

Consuming a regular quantity of food daily as well as using prescribed medicines will significantly improve ones blood glucose management and minimize your chance of diabetes-related risks, such as coronary artery diseases, kidney health problems and nerve impairment. Additionally, eating regularly influences your capability to regulate your weight.

Proteins from lean natural sources can also be very important, specially those which are an excellent source of omega-3 essential fatty acids such as are available in a number of cold water seafood like salmon.

Exercise - This really is encouraged for any individual attempting to lose weight, however it is often especially good for individuals on a diabetic weight reduction program. However, as with anything new, it is very important to monitor ones blood sugar levels just before and after physical exercise in order to ensure you don't overdo it. Doing exercises early in the morning will burn off more calories from fat.

Exercising delivers numerous health and fitness benefits - Strengthening workout routines just like those carried out on fitness equipment at a physical fitness center helps preserve your bones and keep important joints more flexible. Exercise at the same times daily. This can help to promote a more constant blood-sugar level.

Exercise will help you to shed pounds, through building muscle tissue and burning up calories from fat. Of course this may take time, especially to actually spot the differences, each individual activity gets much easier as you become healthier and fitter. Doing exercises regularly to make certain you have got a good level of fitness is essential.

Physical exercise will change fat to more dense, heavier muscle tissue, keeping bodyweight exactly the same yet enhancing cardiac performance and all around health. Supplement the regular exercising with an excellent healthy eating plan.

Type 1 Diabetes is actually a chronic ailment without any cure (as yet), however the outlook on life for individuals managing this disease is far surpassed as compared to 20 years ago. There have been numerous breakthroughs in medication; research and knowledge, decreasing any debilitating problems and increasing the expectations of life on a level to those individuals without type 1diabetes.

Type 1 diabetes is far less frequent compared to type2 diabetes and will also impact on younger people. It's largely seen in men and women younger than 40 and mainly in children below the age of 14.

Type 2 diabetes, however, advances very slowly with no signs or symptoms at all. Regrettably, Type 2 diabetes is generally only identified following the occurrence of a problem, for instance blood circulation problems, nerve damage, eyesight issues, or renal system damage. Type 2 diabetes is treated by diet and physical activity alone or physical activity, tablets and/or insulin.

Picking a beneficial diabetic weight loss diet program is as easy as choosing which tasty recipes you will most surely enjoy. Timing of daily meals is a vital part of a diabetic persons diet program.

Healthy and balanced food options are essential for everybody but for the particular type 2 diabetes sufferers it's significance can't be over-stated. Control over blood glucose levels is of vital significance to prevent the various issues which diabetes could cause. Diabetic healthcare agencies need to interact with patients as advocates and request them to discuss their particular ordeals with other diabetic sufferers.

Research workers identified that extra fat around your stomach contributes to a very much greater risk of health problems such as cardiovascular disease and possibly many forms of cancer. They found that if the majority of your excess fat is within the tummy area, your health problems could be greater compared to if it's elsewhere on your body. Study is however inconsistent as to if it is due exclusively to the menopause or entirely to age group (simply because males as well usually put on weight as they become middle aged), or even a mixture of age and menopause.

Health professionals encourage over weight patients to lose weight as a part of managing their diabetic issues. Adjusting eating habits along with shedding weight might be challenging for some individuals with this ailment. Health care professionals have the means to determine just how much impact a certain carbohydrate foodstuff has on an individual's blood sugar level. This is known as the glycaemic index list.

Health care professionals desire their patients to arrive at a healthy bodyweight just as much as the patient do, therefore it is vital that you interact to achieve that objective. A number of appointments with your health care professional may be required as weight reduction goals progress.

Dietary fiber is very important to a person suffering from diabetes because soluble fiber has a bearing on blood-glucose levels. Dietary fiber food items are not only ideal for colon cleaning, but are additionally a benefit in a weight-reducing program.

Carbohydrate food items, also known as carbs, supply glucose for vitality. Starchy foods, fruits, milk, high fiber vegetables such as corn, and sugars are all carbohydrate foodstuffs. Carbohydrates are generally converted into all kinds of sugar quite early in the digestive function. It is very important to receive a refresher course about carbohydrates and ways to calculate these from your dietician.

Carbohydrates which have very little dietary benefit such as sugary sweet, white-colored breads and also other items created using white flour needs to be excluded. Stick to a straightforward meal plan that delivers uncomplicated, appetizing meals and tasty recipes that will help you take control of your blood sugars. Superior carbohydrates are transformed into glucose by your body, supplying energy for your body.

Exceedingly high amounts of poor carbohydrate consumption bring about higher amounts of blood glucose levels, that impacts on diabetic sufferers drastically. Carbohydrate craving is usually characterized by the lack of ability to stop eating. It's likely you have strong desires for snack foods throughout the day and sweets right after you eat. Incorporating small snack foods of reduced carbohydrates (banana, apple or any negative food stuff) throughout the day can help fill the emptiness in your stomach.

Also a good snacking food is small chicken or turkey pieces, snacking on these every 3 hours during the day is a great aid in maintaining your glucose level.

Low Carbohydrate Diabetic Diet plans could possibly be the most effective plan of action for any dieters that are looking towards shedding weight, as most diabetic diet plans help in retaining blood glucose levels at a good optimum level.

CHAPTER 8
SECRETS TO FINDING THE
BEST DIABETIC RECIPES

Restrictions on a diabetic's diet can make for dull and boring meal options, but that doesn't have to be the case. There are great recipes that offer delicious, healthy meal options for diabetics that the whole family will enjoy!

What to look for in Great Diabetic Recipes

Variety

Great diabetic recipes or diabetic recipes sites will offer a variety of recipes that will provide you with choices for each meal. This will give you options to not get bored with the same recipe and meal night after night.

Nutritional Dietary Information

A good diabetic recipe should provide you with the nutritional information for the finished meal. This is recipe "label reading" just like you would do on any packaged food you pick up in the grocery store.

The important things to watch on the nutritional information are:

Sugar

Carbohydrates

Saturated Fat

The content of the above per serving, should be less than 7 to 9 grams or 20% of your daily intake, generally speaking.

Diabetic Holiday or Specialty Recipes

The easiest time to fall away from healthy eating is during special occasions or Holiday meals. The best diabetic recipe sites will provide holiday diabetic recipes or special event recipes.

There are great Diabetic Thanksgiving Recipes or Christmas Diabetic Recipes that make Holiday cooking for diabetics a healthy event.

Maintaining healthy eating during the Holiday meals and special events is key to overall health. We easily overlook how often a special dinner, birthday or holiday season occurs. These many special days lead to special foods that are usually not on a diabetic diet.

Sticking with healthier meal options on these days is a good way to create a healthy diabetic lifestyle that will carry you to old age.

Not to mention that these holiday meals or special occasions can lead to 5 lbs extra weight gained per year. This will gradually lead to a large increase of weight overtime as you age.

Being overweight is very detrimental to the health of a diabetic.

Knowledgeable Diabetic Tips and Information

The knowledge and care taken with the information on a diabetic recipes site is telling of the true responsibility the site and writers take with the recipes and data they provide.

See what type of data and information the site provides. Is it helpful? Accurate? Or Insightful?

Tools for Managing Diabetes

Good diabetic recipe sites will also provide information or links to tools that aid diabetics in successfully managing their diabetes. This may include books, references, cooking tools, recipes, knowledgeable resources, etc.

Diabetic Recipes to Stay Away From

Use common sense when picking from some so called "diabetic recipes". Things to watch out for are recipes containing:

Sugar or sugary ingredients

Canned fruits or preserves

Anything with "candied" in the title of the recipe (no brainer right)

CHAPTER 9
DIABETICS-DOES A KETO DIET HELP LOWER BLOOD SUGAR LEVELS

Ketogenic diets have been in use since 1924 in pediatrics as a treatment for epilepsy. A ketogenic (keto) diet is one that is high in fat and low in carbs. The design of the ketogenic diet is to shifts the body's metabolic fuel from burning carbohydrates to fats. With the keto diet, the body metabolizes fat, instead of sugar, into energy. Ketones are a byproduct of that process.

Over the years, ketogenic diets have been used to treat diabetes. One justification was that it treats diabetes at its root cause by lowering carbohydrate intake leading to lower blood sugar, which in turn, lowers the need for insulin which minimizes insulin resistance and associated metabolic syndrome. In this way, a ketogenic diet may improve blood glucose (sugar) levels while at the same time reducing the need for insulin. This point of view presents keto diets as a much safer and more effective plan than injecting insulin to counteract the consumption of high carbohydrate foods.

A keto diet is actually a very restrictive diet. In the classic keto diet for example, one gets about 80 percent of caloric requirements from fat and 20 percent from proteins and carbohydrates. This is a marked departure from the norm where the body runs on energy from sugar derived from carbohydrate digestion but by severely limiting carbohydrates, the body is forced to use fat instead.

A ketogenic diet requires healthy food intake from beneficial fats, such as coconut oil, grass-pastured butter, organic pastured eggs, avocado, fish such as salmon, cottage cheese, avocado, almond butter and raw nuts (raw pecans and macadamia). People on ketogenic diets avoid all bread, rice, potatoes, pasta, flour, starchy vegetables, and dairy. The diet is low in vitamins, minerals, and nutrients and require supplementation.

Low carbohydrate diet is frequently recommended for people with type 2 diabetes because carbohydrates turn to blood sugar which in large quantities cause blood sugar to spike. Thus, for a diabetic who already has high blood sugar, eating additional sugar producing foods is like courting danger. By switching the focus from sugar to fat, some patients can experience reduced blood sugar.

Changing the body's primary energy source from carbohydrates to fat leaves behind the byproduct of fat metabolism, ketones in the blood. For some diabetic patients, this can be dangerous as a buildup of ketones may create a risk for developing diabetic ketoacidosis (DKA). DKA is a medical emergency requiring the immediate of a physician. DKA signs include consistently high blood sugar, dry mouth, polyuria, nausea, breath that has a fruit-like odor and breathing difficulties. Complications can lead to diabetic coma.

Is a ketogenic diet safe for people who have received a diagnosis of Type 2 diabetes? The food recommended for people with high blood sugar encourages weight loss: a ketogenic diet has high amounts of fat and is low in carbs, so it is mystifying how such a high-fat diet is an option for alleviating high blood sugar.

The ketogenic diet underlines a low intake of carbohydrates and increased consumption of fat and protein. The body then breaks down fat by a process called "ketosis," and produces a source of fuel called ketones. Usually, the diet improves blood sugar levels while decreasing the body's need for insulin. The diet initially was developed for epilepsy treatment, but the kinds of food and the eating pattern it highlights, are being studied for the benefit of those with Type 2 diabetes.

The ketogenic diet contains foods such as...

pasta,

fruits, and

bread

as a source of body energy. People with Type 2 diabetes suffer from high and unstable blood sugar levels, and the keto diet helps them by allowing the body to preserve their blood sugar at a low healthy level.

How does a keto diet help many with Type 2 diabetes? In 2016, the Journal of Obesity and Eating Disorders published a review suggesting a keto diet may help people with diabetes by improving their A1c test results, more than a calorie diet.

The ketogenic diet places emphasis on the consumption of more protein and fat, making you feel less hungry and therefore leading to weight loss. Protein and fat take longer to digest than carbohydrates and helps to keep energy levels up.

In a nutshell, the ketogenic diet...

lowers blood sugar,

enhances insulin sensitivity and

promotes less dependency on medications.

The Keto Diet Plan. Ketogenic diets are stringent, but if adhered to correctly they can provide a nourishing and healthful nutrition routine. It is about staying away from carbohydrate foods likely to spike blood sugar levels.

People with Type 2 diabetes are often advised to focus on this diet plan as it consists of a mix of low carbohydrate foods, high-fat content, and moderate protein. It is also important because it avoids high-processed foods and indulges in lightly processed and healthy foods.

A ketogenic diet should consist of these types of food...

low-carb vegetables: eat vegetables with every meal. Avoid starchy vegetables like corn and potatoes.

eggs: they contain a low amount of carbohydrates and are a high source of protein.

meats: eat fatty meats but avoid excessive amounts.

High amounts of protein plus low carbohydrates can lead to the liver converting protein into glucose, thus causing the person to come out of ketosis.

fish: an excellent source of protein.

Eat from healthy sources of fat like avocados, seeds, nuts, and olive oil.

It is helpful to go by what your body requires rather than what you feel you need. Always follow your doctor's advice on nutrition and medications and check with him/her before starting a new eating plan.

Although managing your disease can be very challenging, diabetes is not a condition you must just live with. You can make simple changes to your daily routine and lower both your weight and your blood sugar levels. Hang in there, the longer you do it, the easier it gets.

If you are someone who likes going on a lower carbohydrate diet plan to control your blood sugar levels better and see faster rates of weight loss, you might be interested in considering a diet plan called the targeted ketogenic diet.

If you are not familiar with the ketogenic diet plan, this is a very low carbohydrate diet that contains just 5% of the total calories coming from carbohydrates. The remaining calories come from protein at 30% and dietary fat at 65%. Altogether these put you into a state called ketosis, where your body is running off an alternative fuel source.

The problem with this type of diet, however, apart

from the fact it is tough to maintain, is you cannot perform any intense exercise while using it because you are not supplying the number of carbohydrates necessary to do so. On top of that, food cravings are highly probable because let us face it; it is difficult to eat a no-carb diet. You likely love your carbohydrates and cutting them out altogether is not going to be easy.

Nutritional deficiencies can result from this approach. Many of the world's most nutritious foods are carbohydrates - fruits and vegetables, and even these are limited on this diet.

Enter The Targeted Ketogenic Diet. What is the targeted ketogenic diet all about? On this diet plan, you will be doing things a bit differently. Rather than keeping your carbohydrate intake low at all times, you are going to increase your carbohydrate intake adding more carbs to your diet around the times you are active. Doing this will give your body the fuel you need to complete the exercise training, while also ensuring you can still maintain a good nutritional intake. As long as you choose nutritiously dense foods when selecting those carbohydrates, you should have no problem meeting your nutrient needs.

How many carbohydrates you add during this time will depend on your goals...

the amount of exercise you are doing, and

the intensity,

so note it is variable. However, most people will easily be able to get away with 25 to 50 grams of carbohydrates before the workout and another 25 to 50 grams after the session. Potentially, this will give you 400 calories of carbohydrates to play with, so feast on nutrient-dense foods like...

sweet potatoes,

beans,

oats,

fruits, and

vegetables.

If you are interested in the ketogenic diet but do not want to do a full blown ketogenic diet, definitely consider this approach. It may just be the best thing for you.

Although managing your disease can be very challenging, Type 2 diabetes is not a condition you must just live with. You can make simple changes to your daily routine and lower both your weight and your blood sugar levels. Hang in there, the longer you do it, the easier it gets.

CHAPTER 10
SHOULD YOU USE A
KETOGENIC DIET PLAN?

When using a ketogenic diet, your body becomes more of a fat-burner than a carbohydrate-dependent machine. Several researches have linked the consumption of increased amounts of carbohydrates to development of several disorders such as diabetes and insulin resistance.

By nature, carbohydrates are easily absorbable and therefore can be also be easily stored by the body. Digestion of carbohydrates starts right from the moment you put them into your mouth.

As soon as you begin chewing them, amylase (the enzymes that digest carbohydrate) in your saliva is already at work acting on the carbohydrate-containing food.

In the stomach, carbohydrates are further broken down. When they get into the small intestines, they are then absorbed into the bloodstream. On getting to the bloodstream, carbohydrates generally increase the blood sugar level.

This increase in blood sugar level stimulates the immediate release of insulin into the bloodstream. The higher the increase in blood sugar levels, the more the amount of insulin that is release.

Insulin is a hormone that causes excess sugar in the bloodstream to be removed in order to lower the blood sugar level. Insulin takes the sugar and carbohydrate that you eat and stores them either as glycogen in muscle tissues or as fat in adipose tissue for future use as energy.

However, the body can develop what is known as insulin resistance when it is continuously exposed to such high amounts of glucose in the bloodstream. This scenario can easily cause obesity as the body tends to quickly store any excess amount of glucose. Health conditions such as diabetes and cardiovascular disease can also result from this condition.

Keto diets are low in carbohydrate and high in fat and have been associated with reducing and improving several health conditions.

As someone who is working hard to control or prevent Type 2 diabetes, one diet you may have heard about is the ketogenic or keto diet plan. This diet is a very low carbohydrate diet plan consisting of around...

5% total carbohydrates,

30% protein, and a

whopping 65% dietary fat.

If there is one thing this diet will do, its help to control your blood sugar levels. This said, there is more to eating well than just controlling your blood sugar.

Let's go over some of the main reasons why this diet doesn't always stack up to be as great as it sounds...

1. You'll Be Lacking Dietary Fiber. The first big problem with the ketogenic diet is you'll be seriously lacking in dietary fiber. Almost all vegetables are cut from this plan (apart from the very low-carb varieties), and fruits are definitely not permitted. High fiber grains are also out of the equation, so this leaves you with primarily protein and fats - two foods containing no fiber at all.

Go on this diet and you'll find you start to feel backed up in no time.

2. You'll Be Low In Energy. Another big issue with the ketogenic diet is you'll be low in energy to carry out your exercise program. Your body can only utilize glucose as a fuel source for very intense exercise and if you aren't taking in carbohydrates, you'll have no glucose available.

Therefore, the ketogenic diet is not for anyone who wants to lead an active lifestyle with regular workout sessions.

3. You May Suffer Brain Fog. Those who are using the ketogenic diet may also find they suffer from brain fog. Again, this is thanks to the fact your brain primarily runs off glucose.

Some people may find after a week or two of using the diet they start to feel better as their brain can switch over to using ketone bodies as a fuel source, but others may never find they begin to feel better.

All in all, this diet simply does not work for some people for this very reason.

4. Your Antioxidant Status Will Decline. Finally, the last issue with the ketogenic diet is due to the lack of fruit and vegetable content - your antioxidant status is going to sharply decline.

Antioxidants are important for fending off free radical damage, so this isn't something to take lightly. If you aren't taking them in, you could end up ill in the future.

So keep these points in mind as the diet comes with some risks. The ketogenic diet converts fat instead of sugar into energy. It was first created as a treatment for epilepsy but now the effects of the diet are being looked at to help Type 2 diabetics lower their blood sugar. Make sure you discuss the diet with your doctor before making any dietary changes.

Low carb Diet for diabetes

Living with diabetes does not have to mean feeling deprived. People can learn to balance meals and make healthful food choices while still including the foods they enjoy.

Both sugary and starchy carbohydrates can raise blood sugar levels, but people can choose to include these foods in the right portions as part of a balanced meal plan.

For those with diabetes, it is important to monitor the total amount of carbohydrates in a meal. Carbohydrate needs will vary based on many factors, including a person's activity levels and medications, such as insulin.

A dietitian can recommend specific carbohydrate

guidelines to best meet a person's needs. However, as a general rule, people should try to follow the Academy of Nutrition and Dietetics' MyPlate guidelines and include no more than a quarter plate of starchy carbs in one meal.

For people who have diabetes, the key to a beneficial diet, according to the American Diabetes Association (ADA), is as follows:

Include fruits and vegetables.

Eat lean protein.

Choose foods with less added sugar.

Avoid trans fats.

Below is a list of some fruits, vegetables, and foods with less added sugar.

1. Green leafy vegetables

Green leafy vegetables are packed full of essential vitamins, minerals, and nutrients. They also have minimal impact on blood sugar levels.

Leafy greens, including spinach and kale, are a key plant-based source of potassium, vitamin A, and calcium. They also provide protein and fiber.

Some researchers say that eating green leafy vegetables is helpful for people with diabetes due to their high antioxidant content and starch-digesting enzymes.

Green leafy vegetables include:

spinach

collard greens

kale

cabbage

bok choy

broccoli

One small-scale study suggested that kale juice may help regulate blood sugar levels and improve blood pressure in people with subclinical hypertension. In the study, people drank 300 milliliters of kale juice per day for 6 weeks.

People can include green leafy vegetables in their diet in salads, side dishes, soups, and dinners. Combine them with a source of lean protein, such as chicken or tofu.

2. Whole grains

Whole grains contain high levels of fiber and more nutrients than refined white grains.

Eating a diet high in fiber is important for people with diabetes because fiber slows down the digestion process. A slower absorption of nutrients helps keep blood sugar levels stable.

Whole wheat and whole grains are lower on the glycemic index (GI) scale than white breads and rice. This means that they have less of an impact on blood sugar.

Good examples of whole grains to include in the diet are:

brown rice

whole-grain bread

whole-grain pasta

buckwheat

quinoa

millet

bulgur

rye

People can swap white bread or white pasta for whole-grain options.

3. Fatty fish

Fatty fish is a healthful addition to any diet. Fatty fish contains important omega-3 fatty acids called eicosapentaenoic acid (EPA) and docosahexaenoic acid (DHA).

People need a certain amount of healthful fats to keep their body functioning and to promote heart and brain health.

The ADA report that a diet high in polyunsaturated and monounsaturated fats can improve blood sugar control and blood lipids in people with diabetes.

Certain fish are a rich source of both polyunsaturated and monounsaturated fats. These are:

salmon

mackerel

sardines

albacore tuna

herring

trout

People can eat seaweed, such as kelp and spirulina, as plant-based alternative sources of these fatty acids.

Instead of fried fish, which contains saturated and trans fats, people can try baked, roasted, or grilled fish. Pair with a mix of vegetables for a healthful meal choice.

4. Beans

Beans are an excellent food option for people with diabetes. They are source of plant-based protein, and they can satisfy the appetite while helping people reduce their carbohydrate intake.

Beans are also low on the GI scale and are better for blood sugar regulation than many other starchy foods.

Also, beans may help people manage their blood sugar levels. They are a complex carbohydrate, so the body digests them slower than it does other carbohydrates.

Eating beans can also help with weight loss and could help regulate a person's blood pressure and cholesterol.

There is a wide range of beans for people to choose from, including:

kidney beans

pinto beans

black beans

navy beans

adzuki beans

These beans also contain important nutrients, including iron, potassium, and magnesium.

Beans are a highly versatile food choice. People can include a variety of beans in a chili or stew, or in tortilla wraps with salad.

When using canned beans, be sure to choose an option with no added salt. Otherwise, drain and rinse the beans to remove any added salt.

5. Walnuts

Nuts are another excellent addition to the diet. Like fish, nuts contain healthful fatty acids that help keep the heart healthy.

Walnuts are especially high in omega-3 fatty acids called alpha-lipoic acid (ALA). Like other omega-3s, ALA is important for good heart health.

People with diabetes may have a higher risk of heart disease or stroke, so it is important to get these fatty acids through the diet.

A study from 2018 suggested that eating walnuts is linked with a lower incidence of diabetes.

Walnuts also provide key nutrients, such as protein, vitamin B-6, magnesium, and iron.

People can add a handful of walnuts to their breakfast or to a mixed salad.

6. Citrus fruits

Research has shown that citrus fruits, such as oranges, grapefruits, and lemons, have antidiabetic effects.

Eating citrus fruits is a great way to get vitamins and minerals from fruit without the carbohydrates.

Some researchers believe that two bioflavonoid antioxidants, called hesperidin and naringin, are responsible for the antidiabetic effects of oranges.

Citrus fruits are also a great source of:

vitamin C

folate

potassium

7. Berries

Berries are full of antioxidants, which can help prevent oxidative stress. Oxidative stress is linked with a wide range of health conditions, including heart disease and some cancers.

Studies have found chronic levels of oxidative stress in people with diabetes. Oxidative stress occurs when there is an imbalance between antioxidants and unstable molecules called free radicals in the body.

Blueberries, blackberries, strawberries, and raspberries all contain high levels of antioxidants and fiber. They also contain important other vitamins and minerals, including:

vitamin C

vitamin K

manganese

potassium

People can add fresh berries to their breakfast, eat a handful as a snack, or use frozen berries in a smoothie.

8. Sweet potatoes

Sweet potatoes have a lower GI than white potatoes. This makes them a great alternative for people with diabetes, as they release sugar more slowly and do not raise blood sugar as much.

Sweet potatoes are also a great source of:

fiber

vitamin A

vitamin C

potassium

People can enjoy sweet potatoes in a range of ways, including baked, boiled, roasted, or mashed. For a balanced meal, eat them with a source of lean protein and green leafy vegetables or a salad.

9. Probiotic yogurt

Probiotics are the helpful bacteria that live in the human gut and improve digestion and overall health.

Some research from 2011 suggested that eating probiotic yogurt could improve cholesterol levels in people with type 2 diabetes. This could help lower the risk of heart disease.

One review study suggested that consuming probiotic

foods may reduce inflammation and oxidative stress, as well as increase insulin sensitivity.

People can choose a natural yogurt, such as Greek yogurt, with no added sugar. A probiotic yogurt will contain live and active cultures called Lactobacillus or Bifidobacterium.

People can add berries and nuts to yogurt for a healthful breakfast or dessert.

10. Chia seeds

People often call chia seeds a superfood due to their high antioxidant and omega-3 content. They are also a good source of plant-based protein and fiber.

In one small-scale randomized controlled trial from 2017, people who were overweight and had type 2 diabetes lost more weight after 6 months when they included chia seeds in their diet compared with those who ate an oat bran alternative.

The researchers therefore believe that chia seeds can help people manage type 2 diabetes.

People can sprinkle chia seeds over breakfast or salads, use them in baking, or add water to make a dessert.

Foods to limit

One way to manage diabetes with diet is to balance high- and low-GI foods. High-GI foods increase blood sugar more than low-GI foods.

When choosing high-GI foods, limit the portions and pair these foods with protein or healthful fat to reduce the impact on blood sugar and feel full for longer.

Foods high on the GI scale include:

white bread

puffed rice

white rice

white pasta

white potatoes

pumpkin

popcorn

melons

pineapple

People with diabetes may wish to limit or balance the following foods:

Carb-heavy foods

Carbohydrates are an important part of all meals. However, people with diabetes will benefit from limiting their carbohydrate intake in a balanced diet or pairing carbs with a healthful protein or fat source.

High-GI fruits

Most fruits are low on the GI scale, though melons and pineapple are high-GI. This means that they can increase blood glucose more.

Saturated and trans fats

Unhealthful fats, such as saturated and trans fats, can make a person with diabetes feel worse. Many fried and processed foods, including fries, chips, and baked goods, contain these types of fats.

Refined sugar

People with diabetes should aim to limit or avoid refined sugar, likely present in both store-bought and homemade sweets, cakes, and biscuits.

Per day, the American Heart Association advise consuming no more than 24 grams, or 6 teaspoons, of added sugar for women, and 36 grams, or 9 teaspoons, for men. This does not include naturally occurring sugars from foods such as fruit and plain milk.

Sugary drinks

Drinks that contain a lot of sugar, such as energy drinks, some coffees, and shakes, can imbalance a person's insulin levels.

Salty foods

Foods that are high in salt can raise blood pressure. Salt may also appear as sodium on a food label.

The ADA recommend that people keep their daily sodium intake to under 2,300 milligrams per day, which is the same as the recommendation for the general population.

Alcohol

Drinking alcohol in moderation should not have serious risks for people with diabetes and should not affect long-term glucose control.

People using insulin or insulin secretagogue therapies may have a higher risk of hypoglycemia linked to alcohol consumption.

For people who have diabetes and those who do not, the Centers for Disease Control and Prevention (CDC) recommend up to one drink per day for women and up to two drinks per day for men.

A BETTER DIABETIC MEAL PLAN

Meal plans which emphasize fats and proteins do a better job of controlling blood sugar. This is exactly what a ketogenic diet plan offers. An example of a meal which would help a diabetic stabilize and control blood sugar and insulin might be:

2 cups of sauteed squash

2 tablespoons of butter

5 ounces of grilled sirloin steak

1 peach for dessert

Total calories for this meal would work out to 610.5

and the caloric ratio of "carbohydrate:protein:fat" would be 16% carbs, 25% protein and 60% fat.

According to the more than 50 studies done on the effects of ketogenic diets on diabetic and non diabetic health, this ratio of fat and protein to carbohydrate intake would keep the blood glucose levels well under 130 mg/dl. And most importantly, ketogenic meals taste better and do a better job of satisfying hunger. These factors which would help the patient stick to the diet, and consistently control blood sugar and insulin to healthy levels.

Diabetic Meal Plan Example for a Day

Here's a full day's menu of examples of diabetic meal plans that can be enjoyed on a ketogenic diet:

Breakfast (427 calories, 71% fat, 22% protein, 4% carb)

 1 slice of Cheese and Onion Quiche

 Coffee with cream

Lunch (789 calories, 71% fat, 20% protein, 9% carb)

 1 cup of steamed broccoli with 1 tablespoon butter

 2 tablespoons of creamy hollandaise sauce

 8 ounces of herb baked salmon

 1/2 cup of blueberries with 1 oz cream

Dinner (876 calories, 78% fat, 15% protein, 7% carb)

 6 ounces Low Carb Meatloaf

1 cup steamed cauliflower with 1 tablespoon butter

1 cup Low Carb Cole Slaw

Bedtime Snack

Creamy Chocolate Milk

Meal 1 – Keto Egg Muffins

Ingredients:

4 cherry tomatoes

¼ cup red onion, chopped

1 cup mixed greens (Spinach is great too!)

8 egg yolks

⅓ cup bacon, crumbled

1 ⅕ cup cheddar cheese, shredded

3 tbsp. unsweetened almond milk (optional)

½ tsp garlic salt

Instructions:

Preheat the oven to 400°F (200°C).

Separate the egg yolks from the whites into a large mixing bowl. Discard or save the egg whites for another occasion.

Wash and finely chop the mixed greens, tomatoes, and onion. Add to the egg yolk mixture.

Add bacon, cheese, unsweetened almond milk, and garlic salt to the large mixing bowl with the veggies (personal recommendation: Keep out about 3 tbsps. of cheese to sprinkle on top once muffins have baked). Mix well.

Grease the muffin tin with oil and pour a ¼ cup + 1 tbsp. of the egg mixture evenly into the muffin slots, which should yield 6 muffins. NOTE: You can use muffin cups to line the muffins to save time during clean up.

Pop the muffin tray into the oven for about 12 minutes or until the edges are slightly a toasty brown.

Immediately after taking the egg muffins out of the muffin tin, sprinkle tops of muffins with remaining cheese.

Let cool for 2 minutes before serving.

Meal 2 – Keto Cobb Salad

Ingredients:

4 cherry tomatoes

½ avocado

1 hardboiled egg

2 cups mixed green salad

2 oz. chicken, shredded

1 oz. feta cheese, crumbled,

¼ cup bacon, crumbled

Instructions:

Dice the tomatoes and avocado, and slice the hardboiled egg.

Place 2 cups of mixed green salad into a large salad bowl or plate.

Measure out 2 oz. chicken, 1 oz. feta cheese, and ¼ cup bacon.

Place tomatoes, avocado, egg, chicken, feta, and bacon in horizontal rows on top of the mixed greens.

OPTIONAL: You can add 1 tbsp. of Ranch dressing for 73 calories and about 8 grams of fat (NOT included in the nutrition facts).

Enjoy the whole serving.

Meal 3 – Pepperoni Pizza Bites

Ingredients:

6 Slices (34 g), sandwich sliced pepperoni

2 tbsp. pizza sauce

3 oz. fresh mozzarella

1 tbsp. fresh oregano

Instructions:

Preheat the oven to 400 F (200 C). Using kitchen scissors, snip three ½-inch cuts around the edges of each pepperoni slice, leaving the center uncut (like a 3-leaf clover).

Press each pepperoni slice down into a regular sized muffin pant. Bake slices for 5 minutes, until edges are slightly crispy, but still bright red. Remove from oven, and let the slices cool in pans to harden (this helps the bites hold their shape).

As pepperoni cups are cooking, finely dice fresh oregano.

To remove excess oil, after the bites have cooked, place them on a paper towel for about 10 seconds.

Wipe the grease out of the muffin pan with a paper towel, then return the cups to the pan. Place ½ tsp. of pizza sauce then ½ of an oz. of mozzarella in each cup. Sprinkle with fresh oregano.

Place bites back in the oven for 3 minutes, or just until the cheese melts.

Allow pepperoni bites to cool for about 3-5 minutes.

Meal 4 – Chocolate Keto Fat Bombs

Ingredients:

¼ cup unsweetened cocoa powder (or cacao powder)

5 tbsp. natural chunky peanut butter

6 tbsp. shelled hemp seeds

½ cup, coconut oil

2 tbsp. 10% heavy cream

1 tsp. vanilla extract

2 tbsp. Stevia

4 tbsp. unsweetened coconut flakes

Instructions:

Mix together cocoa powder, peanut butter, and hemp seeds in a large bowl.

Add room temp coconut oil and mix until it becomes a paste.

Add cream, vanilla, and stevia and mix until it becomes a paste again.

Roll into balls. You should be able to make about 12 balls total, which equals 6 servings (2 balls = 1 serving).

Roll into shredded coconut (coconut included in nutrition facts, but optional if you are not a fan).

Place balls on parchment paper on a baking tray.

Freeze for 10 minutes.

CONCLUSION

According to medical studies, obesity and weight gain can greatly increase the risk for diabetes and cardiovascular diseases. It can also have negative impacts on those already diagnosed with Type 2 diabetes, aggravating glycemic control and insulin levels. Therefore, the American Heart Association recommends individuals suffering from diabetes or at risk for diabetes to aim for a BMI of 25 kg/m or lower. They suggest healthy weight loss may be the most important way to manage Type 2 diabetes.

Diabetes and Weight

Based on studies, the American Heart Association states that diabetes and obesity are interlinked conditions. Many cases of diabetes have been shown to be caused by obesity or rapid weight gain in individuals with insulin resistance. Insulin resistance is caused by the body becoming numbed by rapid spikes in blood sugar levels due to diets rich in sugars, unhealthy fats and refined carbohydrates. When these types of diets are not modified when an individual's body becomes insulin resistant, it can quickly lead to Type 2 diabetes.

When an individual has diabetes, their metabolism cannot handle blood sugar levels, leading to too much glucose and cholesterol in the blood. The excess glucose can quickly lead to weight gain. When insulin injections are added into the equation, more glucose is added into the blood. This can easily lead to further weight gain. In return, the weight gain can aggravate blood sugar levels, leading to an unfortunate circular pattern.

Therefore, it is very important for diabetic individuals to work toward weight control in order to prevent further complications with their diabetes that may lead to cardiovascular diseases. This can be accomplished with a diet that avoids refined carbohydrates and is rich in vitamins and minerals combined with a regular fitness program. Your doctor or a health expert will have suggestions on the best weight loss regime for you to undertake.

Weight Loss Benefits

There are many benefits of weight loss in diabetic individuals, including lowering blood sugar levels as stated above. Since diabetes is linked with weight gain and loss, when you begin to shed pounds, blood sugar levels should begin to lower as well. If you are successful with your weight loss program, there is the chance that you will be able to stop taking your insulin medication. Since weight loss can lead to controlled blood sugar levels, you may no longer need the medication in order to stabilize it, especially if the condition has been caused by obesity or rapid weight gain.

Weight loss will also lead to a reduction of blood pressure and to lower cholesterol levels. This aids in preventing the complications that could lead to cardiovascular diseases. The combination of lower blood sugar levels, lower blood pressure and lower cholesterol levels will not only prevent complications and the aggravation of diabetes, but it will lead to a much healthier body and will generally improve your way of life.

Having a good diet plan is essential to maintaining good health after you have been diagnosed with diabetes. There are many misconceptions on how you will never be able to eat again after the diagnosis and that is not true and what must be kept in mind is a diet that will help you maintain the correct sugar levels in your blood. If you maintain a good sugar level then you can prevent the damage that can be caused by diabetes.

When looking for a diet that is best for you and one that limits the amount of sugar and carbohydrates is best. Keep in mind that the carbohydrates you eat turn into sugar once they are digested into your blood stream. When you are looking for the foods that are good for you then loos at food that are grown because these are an excellent source of nutrition. Starches in the form of wholegrain cereals and bread should be included in your diet. Healthy proteins is also very essential.

Maintaining a healthy weight is also very important and this is best accomplished by a healthy diet and a regimented exercise program. A good diet along with exercise will help to control your sugar to safe levels. Smoking and alcohol are not recommended when you are working to maintain a healthy diabetic lifestyle. A person can life a full and healthy lifestyle with diabetes as long as they can control there diet and follow there doctors recommendations.

Just remember that when you have diabetes this is a wake up call to get your health and lifestyle under control and you should know that you can do it.

Each of us probably knows someone who has diabetes. A large chunk of the annual healthcare expenses goes to the treatment and maintenance of diabetes related symptoms and ailments. This is because diabetic people have their own specialized lifestyle.

Medication must be ready all the time, food intake must be kept in moderation and the immune system must be always up. Even if you are a diabetic you can still enjoy your life through moderation and constant discipline. To keep the symptoms of diabetes at bay, here are some simple guidelines:

Know the Types of Workouts That Works

A lot of people assume that diabetics are not healthy enough to exercise. They can do a wide range of exercises that can keep them healthy as long as they are properly monitored. Having a workout buddy is great for diabetics to keep an eye on their condition while in a physical activity. To avoid exercise induced complications, the diabetic person must do works outs that have less risks for injuries such as blisters and bruises. Swimming and water related exercises are great for them because the water lessens the stress in their joints and there are less friction related cuts and blisters.

Stress Management

Diabetic patients must always keep their immune system at its best condition. Because of this, they must

use stress management techniques to lessen the negative effects of stress to the immune system. The right type of stress management must be employed because stress cannot be avoided all the time. Research and do techniques that work for you. Many people find physical activities that don't require too much thinking therapeutic in relieving stress.

Eat Your Meals at the Same Time Each Day

Food intake should be organized for the diabetic patient. It is important for diabetics to eat at the same time each day. Having a schedule will surely help you in making sure that you don't miss a meal. Carrying food for emergencies is a good way of preventing missed meals when you have hectic schedules.

Control the Amount of Food You Eat Per Meal

Binge eating is not an option for diabetic patients. The amount of food that the diabetic eats must be monitored properly. Get a meal buddy to make sure that the amount of food you take in is monitored. Your spouse or your children can also help in keeping the amount of food you are eating monitored.

Keep the Food Type You Consume Balanced

The percentage of fats, protein, and carbohydrates that a diabetic person requires is different from what a non-diabetic person needs. To learn about the right percentage of fats, carbohydrates and proteins in your diet and other symptoms of diabetes information. Also have him or her suggest food items that are recommended for you.

The facts are nine out of 10 people who are newly diagnosed with type 2 diabetes are overweight or obese. It is estimated that over 80% of the tens of millions of individuals who suffer from Type 2 diabetes and pre-diabetes fall into the overweight/obese category. This is one of the main contributors to the developing the disease of diabetes.

So as you might expect controlling your weight is important to controlling diabetes. Every diabetic should focus on slow, intentional weight loss over a period of time. This will decrease your need for insulin and/or improve your body's ability to produce insulin, improve your heart health, improve self-esteem, and make you sexy once again!

By losing those excess pounds you will also reduce their risk factors for developing stroke, heart attack, and retinal damage, kidney failure, along with dozens of other health benefits directly or indirectly related to diabetes.

I know and you know losing weight and keeping it off is as much of a challenge for those who have diabetes as it is for those who don't. If it weren't there wouldn't be thousands of weight loss programs making billions of dollars every year!

As a diabetic it is important that you seek the help of qualified professionals to help you lose the weight. You may require changes in medication and/or other treatments.

I want to clear one thing up here for a second. It is not so much about losing weight as it is about losing body fat!

When you "lose weight", you lose muscle, water, and fat. You should focus on building muscle and losing body fat simultaneously. This is the most effective way to reap those benefits I mentioned earlier.

Losing weight as a diabetic is accomplish the same way that weight loss is achieved under any other circumstance.

Most people think weight loss is about eating fewer calories and burning more calories than eaten, which is partially true. Weight loss is about changing your mindset, changing the make-up of your diet and nutrition habits and throwing in some physical activity.

Weight loss (aka fat loss) of 1-2 pounds a week is a good goal to aim for. Don't be in a rush for that quick fix that I know you are thinking of. Losing 20 pounds in 5 days isn't realistic and it's not healthy by any means (I don't care who told you or where you read it).

The goal of any weight loss program is for gradual and steady weight loss that can be maintained over an extended period time till your end goal is reached, whatever it may be. This will eventually result in a healthy body and mind. Almost all the time this can also result in the elimination of any and all medications required to control your Type 2 diabetes.

Like mentioned earlier, exercise plays an important role in your weight loss success and in controlling your diabetes. There are two main reasons individuals should exercise. First, exercise reduces the body's need for insulin to control blood sugar levels and improves the body's ability to produce insulin to better control blood sugar levels. Second, it increases the body's metabolism, thus allowing individuals to burn body fat easier. Of course there are many other reasons to exercise but those are two of the main ones for diabetics and weight loss.

Here some basic steps to take to guarantee you are on the right path for weight loss and controlling your diabetes.

• Think positive, be optimistic, and set goals- If you keep telling yourself "you'll never lose all this weight" then you won't! Conquer whatever fears and hang-ups you have inside yourself or else you'll end up getting frustrated and quit. Also, without setting any goals you'll never know where you're headed. Be specific-date, exact weight, how you'll feel, what will happen if you don't get there?

• Get some support- therapist, family, close friends, support groups, etc. Weight loss is not easy, sometimes having people to talk and turn too can keep you on track and focused.

• Eliminate any simple sugars- soda, deserts, candy, juice, etc.

• Cut back on complex carbohydrates - pasta, rice, potatoes, corn, bread, etc.

• Make protein foods a majority of your meals- fish, chicken, turkey, beef, seafood, nuts, etc.

• Tons of fiber- vegetables, some fruits (berries), beans, nuts, and supplements (Benefiber, Metamucil, or any other)

• Use healthy fats- olive oil, real butter, Smart Balance, canola oil, coconut oil, fish oil, and any sort of nut oil.

• Drink tons of water- a gallon a day keeps melts the pounds away. Yes, I'm serious!

• Exercise/Physical activity- either short bouts of high intensity exercise (e.g. 30 second sprints with 1 min of rest in between, repeated 10-12 times) or 30-45 minutes of moderate intensity exercise 4-5 times a week. (e.g. weight training, circuit training, cardio mixed with weights, etc.)

• Be consistent- without consistency you will not get the results you are looking for. Consistently control your diet, exercise, stay in a positive state of mind, take to your support team, etc.

Using the tips I laid out above you will be well on your way to successful weight loss, better blood sugars, and a healthier life. Now it's all up to you to take the first step my friend.

Do not go yet; One last thing to do

If you enjoyed this book or found it useful I'd be very grateful if you'd post a short review on it. Your support really does make a difference and I read all the reviews personally so I can get your feedback and make this book even better.

Thanks again for your support!

CPSIA information can be obtained
at www.ICGtesting.com
Printed in the USA
BVHW040802040321
R11947400001B/R119474PG601388BVX00001B/1